Dedication

To the couples who still believe
that love can evolve, not erode.

To every woman who feels unseen and
every man who dares to feel again.

May you find your rhythm, your laughter, and your fire.

Comme on dit en France...
que l'amour se pratique, pas seulement se promet.

As we say in France...
love must be practiced, not just promised.

MAKE AMERICA MATE AGAIN

A Frenchman's Guide to Healing American Bedrooms

BY GUY BLAISE

First Edition – 2025

Printed in the United States of America

For permissions, media inquiries, or interviews:

www.HowToLoveLikeTheFrench.com

Cover design and concept by Guy Blaise

Illustrations by Guy Blaise

ISBN: 979-8-218-74767-1

Disclaimer:
This book is intended for reflection, not diagnosis.

For those in fragile relationships, it may awaken truths that require courage, communication, and sometimes, professional help.

Table of Contents

Introduction

Dear Americans,

I didn't come to America to write about your marriages. Honestly, I thought I'd enjoy your big cars, big houses, and bigger refrigerators. But then I saw something even bigger— your problem in the bedroom.

You have freedom, democracy, and Netflix in every room... yet no one kisses. You argue louder than you touch. You text faster than you caress. You plan vacations better than you plan seduction.

As a Frenchman, this was shocking. In France, we fight about politics at the table—but we still make love after dessert. You? You're filing "sex" somewhere between laundry and dentist appointments.

This book is my love letter and my warning. Marriage is not a contract. It's not a business merger. It's not "roommates with joint custody." It's supposed to be passion, play, fire. You don't need another debate. You need more neck kisses while unloading the dishwasher.

Make America Mate Again is my invitation to put the romance back where it belongs. Because trust me: No country ever collapsed from too much kissing.

Avec provocation et tendresse,
Guy Blaise

DESIRE NEEDS MAINTENANCE, NOT MIRACLES

Dear Americans,

Let's start with a smile. A penis is like a golf ball—it's always looking for a hole. But desire isn't just biology; it's curiosity that never retires. A man in love keeps chasing his partner, not because he must, but because he still wants to. When the spark fades, don't blame age or marriage. Check your health, your laughter, your tenderness. Passion isn't lost; it's neglected. Maintain it like a classic car: polish it, drive it, enjoy the ride.

Comme on dit en France:
Un homme amoureux poursuit sa femme, même après trente ans.

As we say in France:
A man in love still chases his wife, even after thirty years.

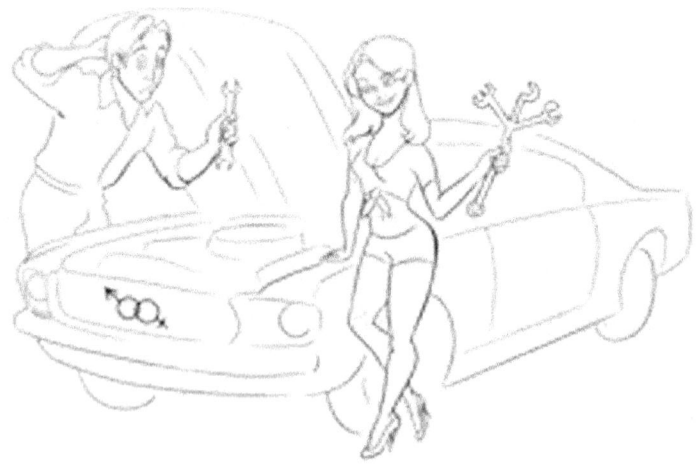

"À quoi penses-tu?"
(What are you thinking about?)

PURITANISM STILL HAUNTS YOUR BEDROOMS

Dear Americans,

Your Puritan roots linger between your sheets. You can build skyscrapers, launch rockets, dissect politics endlessly—but when it comes to sex, you fall silent. You call it "private," but really, it's shame disguised as politeness. Couples avoid the conversation until desire dies quietly in silence. In France, sex isn't a sin—it's art, dialogue, nourishment. We speak of it, laugh about it, study it, honor it. Until you dare to speak freely, intimacy will remain crippled.

Comme on dit en France:
Le silence tue plus de couples que l'infidélité.

As we say in France:
Silence kills more couples than infidelity.

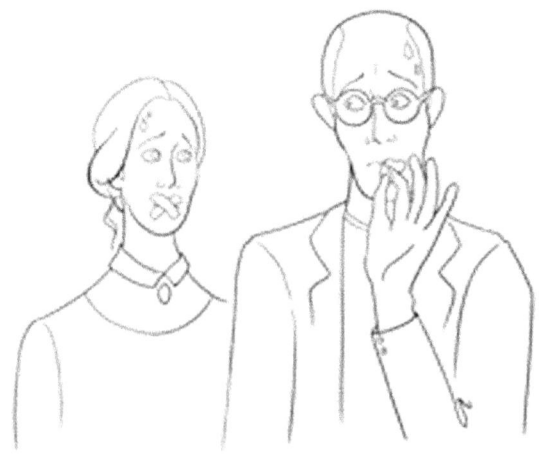

"À quoi penses-tu?"

(What are you thinking about?)

You're Having Sex. But Are You Making Love?

Dear Americans,

Porn has confused you. Too many know how to "fuck," but not how to make love. Fucking is friction; making love is fusion—of bodies, yes, but also of souls. Sex can be routine, a release, an exercise. But love lingers in the tenderness, the slowness, the reverence. Men and women should know the difference, and every couple should make a conscious choice. In France, we know you can fuck without making love, but when you make love… fucking becomes art.

Comme on dit en France:
Le sexe s'oublie. La tendresse reste dans la peau.

As we say in France:
Sex fades, but tenderness lingers in the skin.

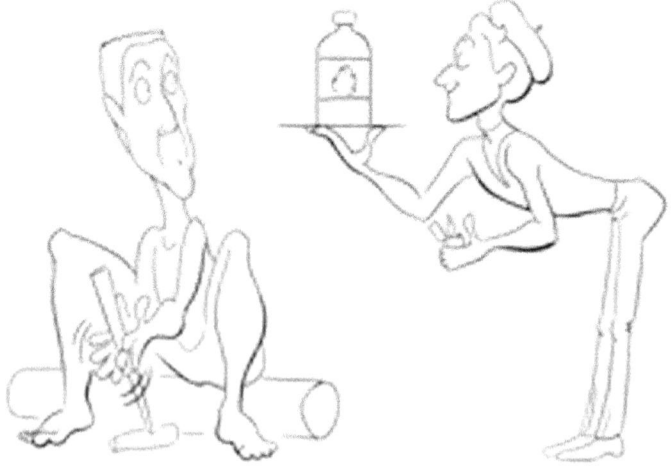

"À quoi penses-tu?"

(What are you thinking about?)

YOUR ORGASM ISN'T THE FINALE. PRESENCE IS.

Dear Americans,

Men often race to the finish line, but women crave the journey. Think of making love like eating your favorite meal—slow down, savor it, enjoy the flavors. Women want to feel desired, not rushed. Held, not hurried. Her climax is not the prize; it's part of the landscape. Desire grows not through speed but through sensation, not through pounding but through presence. For her, fulfillment is not the finale—it's knowing you were truly there, every second.

Comme on dit en France:
Le sommet n'est rien sans la beauté du chemin.

As we say in France:
The peak means nothing without the beauty of the climb.

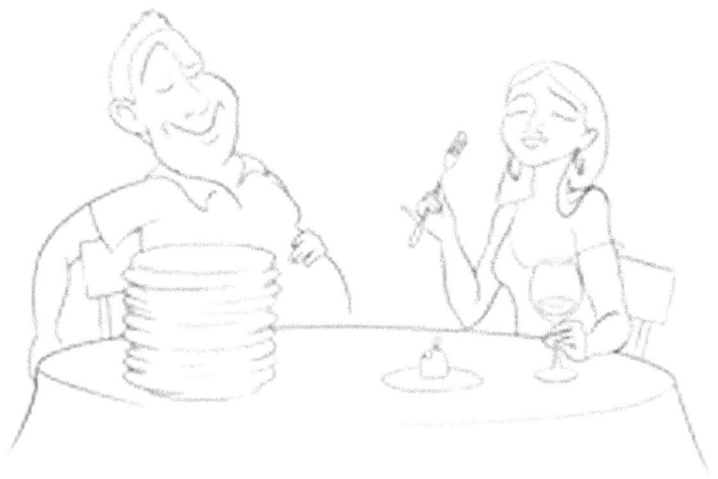

"À quoi penses-tu?"

(What are you thinking about?)

WITHOUT EMOTION, SEX IS JUST SWEAT

Dear Americans,

The body can move. The sheets can wrinkle. But without emotion, it's just exercise. Your wife wants your eyes to linger, your soul to arrive, your presence to burn with her. Without emotion, sex becomes routine—functional, empty. With emotion, even a simple caress becomes unforgettable. Passion isn't performance; it's presence. Desire is not about technique; it's about sincerity. The body responds to touch, but the soul responds to meaning. Without emotion, sex is hollow. With it, love becomes sacred.

Comme on dit en France:
Le corps peut bouger… mais sans l'âme, il ne fait que transpirer.

As we say in France:
The body may move… but without soul, it only sweats.

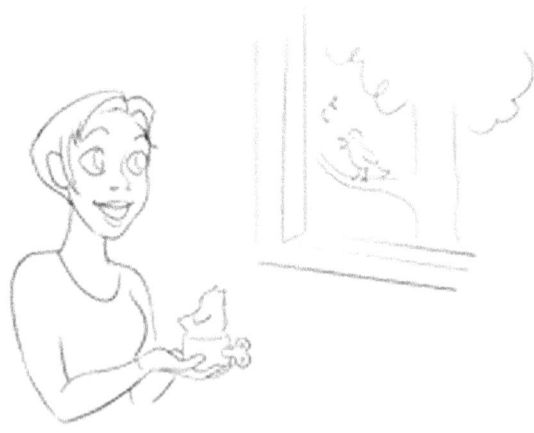

10

"À quoi penses-tu?"
(What are you thinking about?)

IN FRANCE, THE BEDROOM IS NOT A CHORE CHART

Dear Americans,

Keep a bottle of water by your bed—not a checklist. No gold stars, no scorecards, no "Did we do it?" Only: "Did we feel it?" The French know intimacy is never about accomplishment. It's about energy, surrender, curiosity, play. When sex becomes a task, desire suffocates. But when the bed feels like freedom, a woman blooms. Lovers don't keep score—they keep rhythm. If love becomes duty, passion evaporates. If it becomes discovery, it grows endlessly.

Comme on dit en France:
L'amour n'est pas une tâche. C'est une touche.

As we say in France:
Love is not a task. It's a touch.

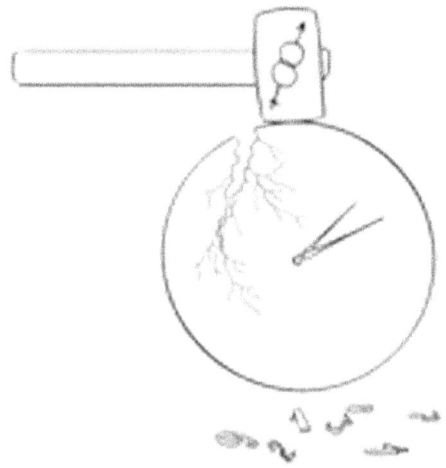

"À quoi penses-tu?"

(What are you thinking about?)

EMOTIONAL FOREPLAY IS EVERYTHING

Dear Americans,

Psychologists once tempted children with candy: wait, and you'll get more. Desire works the same way. Before fingers explore skin, let your eyes explore her soul. Before lips touch, let words melt walls. Women don't bloom from demand—they bloom from devotion. Emotional foreplay is not optional; it's essential. It begins with listening, curiosity, reverence. It's the look that whispers, "I still choose you." Her body opens when her heart feels seen. Seduction is 80 percent soul, 20 percent skin. Neglect the soul, and the body will never surrender.

Comme on dit en France:
La peau s'offre à celui qui sait parler au cœur.

As we say in France:
The skin yields to the one who speaks to the heart.

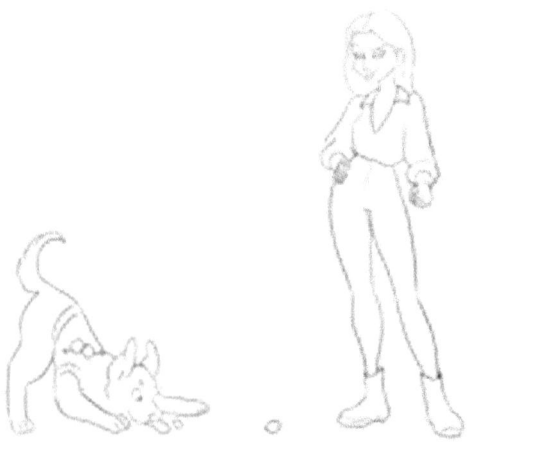
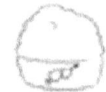

14

"À quoi penses-tu?"

(What are you thinking about?)

Don't Fake What You Don't Feel

Dear Americans,

Couples fake sex when attraction fades. Forced moans, staged orgasms, hollow compliments— performance without sincerity. What a waste of energy! Pretending is poison. Authenticity is magnetic. If you're tired, admit it. If you're hungry for her, show it. She doesn't need perfection—she needs truth. Real intimacy lives in honesty, not acting. When your desire is real, your touch carries fire. And trust me: She will always know the difference.

Comme on dit en France:
Le vrai désir fait le vrai frisson.

As we say in France:
Real desire creates real shivers.

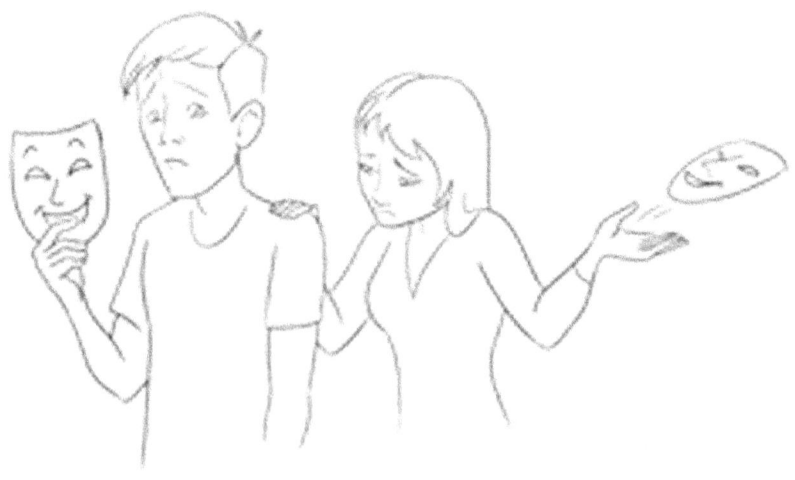

"À quoi penses-tu?"

(What are you thinking about?)

SCHEDULED SEX FEELS LIKE A DENTIST APPOINTMENT

Dear Americans,

It's not that scheduling intimacy is evil, but sex is instinct, not obligation. Early in love, passion flows naturally. Then life piles on kids, bills, deadlines. Couples think penciling it in will solve the drought. But desire doesn't thrive in Outlook reminders. She doesn't crave structure; she craves surprise. No woman wants to be treated like a calendar task. Don't reduce passion to logistics. Don't book her—burn for her. Desire is reborn in spontaneity, in impulse, in the moments you didn't plan.

Comme on dit en France:
On ne fait pas l'amour par obligation, mais par impulsion.

As we say in France:
We don't make love out of obligation, but out of impulse.

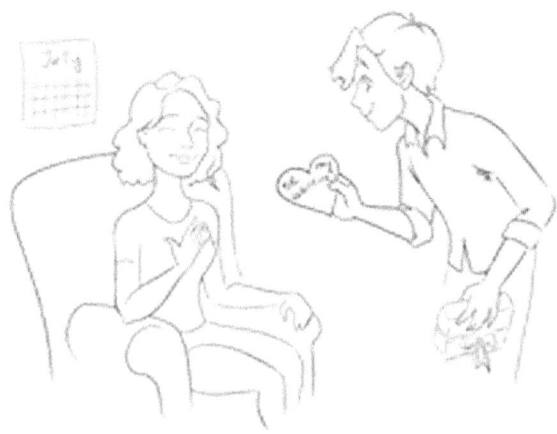

"À quoi penses-tu?"

(What are you thinking about?)

YOU CAN'T FLIP A SWITCH THAT'S BEEN OFF ALL DAY

Dear Americans,

If you've ignored your partner all day, don't expect them to light up like Times Square at bedtime. Passion isn't a light switch; it's more like a fireplace. If you don't add wood (attention, laughter, affection), don't be surprised when there are no flames. You can't walk past your partner like a roommate, then expect them to purr like a lover. By night, they're not cold—just unplugged. Want them to glow? Charge their heart all day. That's how desire works.

Comme on dit en France:
Quand le cœur s'est éteint, aucune étincelle ne suffit—
il faut rallumer le soleil.

As we say in France:
Once the heart goes dark, no spark will do—
you must bring the sun back.

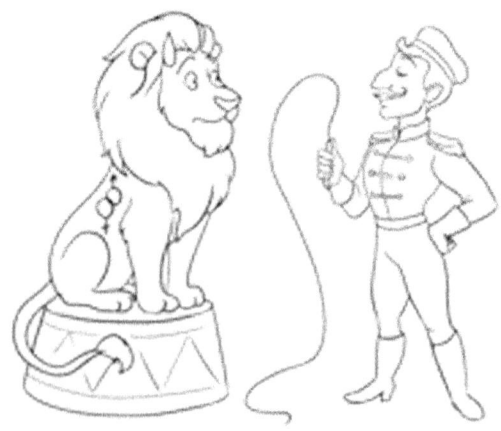

20

"À quoi penses-tu?"

(What are you thinking about?)

COMPLIMENT SOMETHING NON-SEXUAL

Dear Americans,

A sincere compliment won't kill anyone, yet too many men reserve admiration for the bedroom. Desire doesn't only grow from attraction—it grows from appreciation. Don't just praise curves; praise character. Tell your partner she's brilliant, hilarious, resilient. Notice how she parents, how she solves problems, how her mind lights up a room. Admiration for essence—not just appearance—builds intimacy. A woman adored for her spirit will offer her body more freely than one reduced to it.

Comme on dit en France:
Le désir commence quand elle se sent admirée,
pas seulement déshabillée.

As we say in France:
Desire begins when she feels admired—not just undressed.

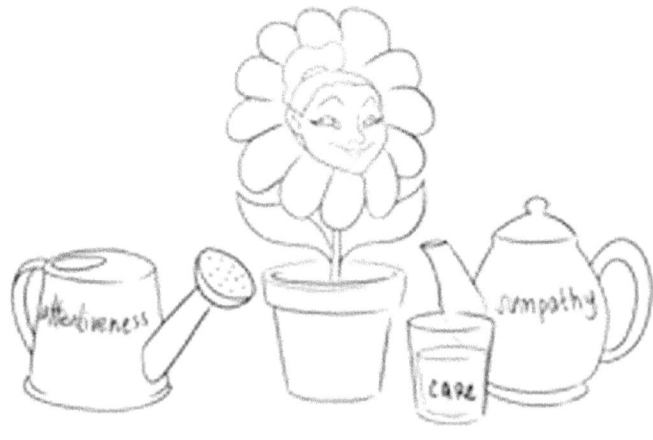

"À quoi penses-tu?"

(What are you thinking about?)

SAFETY IS
THE REAL APHRODISIAC

Dear Americans,

Sex begins in the mind. If your partner feels unsafe, no candle, playlist, or lingerie will matter. An anxious heart cannot surrender. True passion is born when she knows you won't rush her, won't judge her, won't disappear. Safety isn't boring. It's the spark that ignites every fire. With safety, even silence becomes seductive; without it, touch is just mechanics. Give her peace, and she'll give you passion. Emotional security is not the enemy of desire—it's the fuel.

Comme on dit en France:
Une femme rassurée, c'est une femme qui s'ouvre.

As we say in France:
A woman who feels safe is a woman who opens.

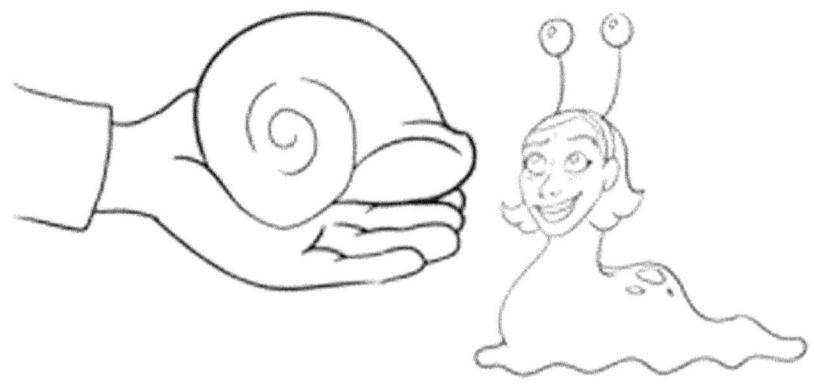

"À quoi penses-tu?"
(What are you thinking about?)

"I SEE YOU" IS MORE POWERFUL THAN "I WANT YOU"

Dear Americans,

Telling your partner "I want you" is flattering, but "I see you" transforms everything. Desire without recognition feels hollow. When your partner feels truly seen—her thoughts, her struggles, her essence—she feels safe. And safety is the soil where passion blooms. Lust without presence is shallow; admiration without depth is fleeting. But when your gaze reaches beyond her body into her being, she ignites. She becomes flame—not because you demanded fire, but because you honored her existence. Husbands, if you can't see your partner, call an eye doctor. It's the most urgent vision check you'll ever need.

Comme on dit en France:
Quand une femme se sent vue, elle devient flamme.

As we say in France:
When a woman feels seen, she becomes flame.

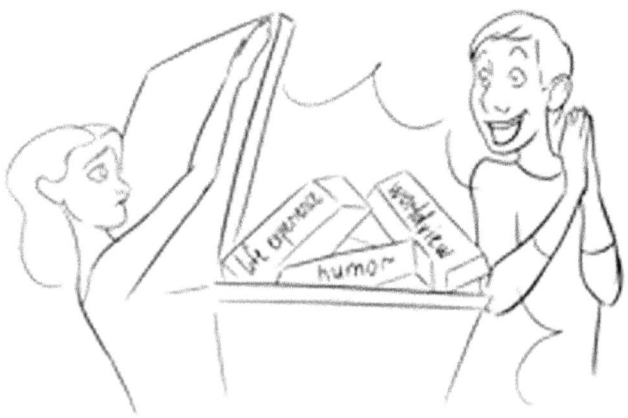

"À quoi penses-tu?"

(What are you thinking about?)

RESENTMENT LIVES WHERE CONNECTION IS STARVED

Dear Americans,

A sexless relationship is not always the husband's fault—sometimes it begins with the wife. But truthfully, a sexless marriage rarely starts in the bedroom; it starts in the heart. When connection dries up, resentment creeps in quietly. Each ignored emotion, each unspoken slight, builds distance. A body won't yield when the spirit feels abandoned. Neglect makes desire brittle. Silence stiffens intimacy. The cure is not technique, but tenderness. Patience, affection, care—these reopen the heart. And when the heart reopens, the body follows. Desire is not mechanical. Fix the fracture, and passion blooms again.

Comme on dit en France:
Là où le cœur se ferme, le corps s'éteint.

As we say in France:
Where the heart shuts down, the body shuts off.

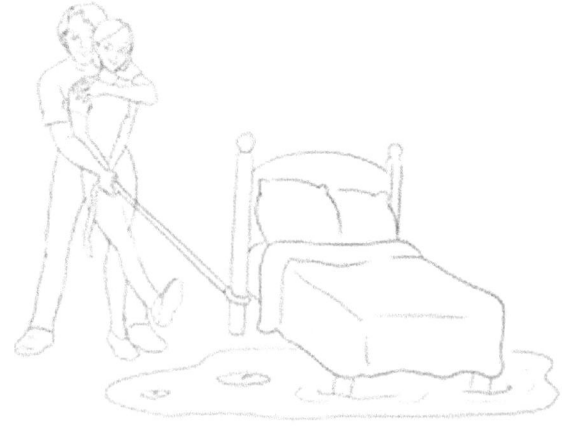

28

"À quoi penses-tu?"

(What are you thinking about?)

DESIRE DOESN'T LIVE IN OVERWHELM

Dear Americans,

I've never seen women juggle so much—five calendars, a weather report, three kids' lunches, and somehow, your dry cleaning. And you wonder why she's not thinking about lingerie? She's not cold—she's cooked. Passion doesn't bloom in chaos; it suffocates there. If you want fire, stop piling wood on her back. Fold laundry. Order dinner. Tell a joke. Give her five minutes to exhale, and maybe she'll remember you exist. Desire isn't lazy; it's buried under your to-do list.

Comme on dit en France:
Une femme surchargée n'a pas le luxe du désir.

As we say in France:
An overloaded woman doesn't have the luxury of desire.

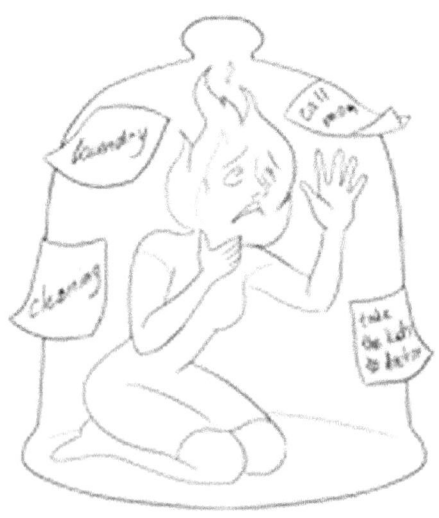

"À quoi penses-tu?"

(What are you thinking about?)

SHE CAN'T RELAX
IF SHE'S MANAGING EVERYTHING

Dear Americans,

You want her to melt into your arms, but her brain is sprinting an Olympic marathon: dentist, bills, laundry, "what to get your mother." She's not resisting you—she's resisting insanity. Desire needs surrender, but who can surrender while running a mental spreadsheet at midnight? If she's carrying everything, she has nothing left for you. Want her body to relax? Start by relaxing her mind. Do the damn dishes. Book the appointment. Suddenly, her shoulders drop—and maybe her clothes, too.

Comme on dit en France:
Si elle pense à tout, elle ne pensera jamais à toi.

As we say in France:
If she's thinking of everything, she won't have space to think of you.

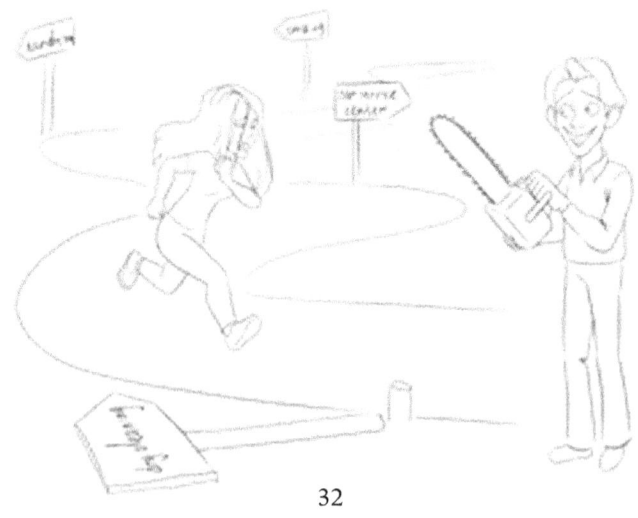

"À quoi penses-tu?"

(What are you thinking about?)

DESIRE ISN'T A SWITCH. IT'S SPACE.

Dear Americans,

You think you can ignore her all day, then flip a switch like Alexa: "Sexy mode on." Désolé, it doesn't work like that. Desire isn't electricity; it's atmosphere. If her head has been full of unpaid labor—logistics, emails, emotional babysitting—there's no room for passion. You can't demand desire; you must build space for it. Clear her plate, pour her wine, make her laugh. Give her the rarest gift in America: a quiet mind. That's when intimacy has a chance to exhale.

Comme on dit en France:
Le désir a besoin de vide pour respirer.

As we say in France:
Desire needs space to breathe.

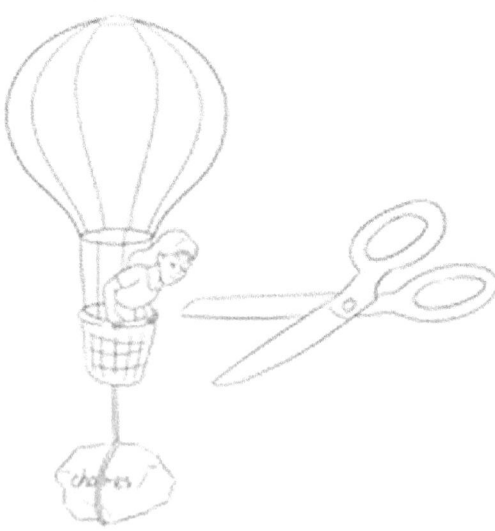

"À quoi penses-tu?"

(What are you thinking about?)

You Want a Lover?
Then Don't Treat Her
Like Your Assistant

Dear Americans,

Some of you treat your wives like unpaid interns: "Did you book my appointment? Pay the bill? Order my socks?" Then you expect her to dress like a lover at night? Non, monsieur. Desire doesn't grow in Excel sheets. A woman doesn't want to be your secretary—she wants to be your equal. If you want passion, stop delegating and start participating. Initiative is foreplay. Nothing is sexier than a man who handles his own damn calendar. Only then does romance have oxygen.

Comme on dit en France:
Une amante n'est pas une secrétaire.

As we say in France:
A lover is not a secretary.

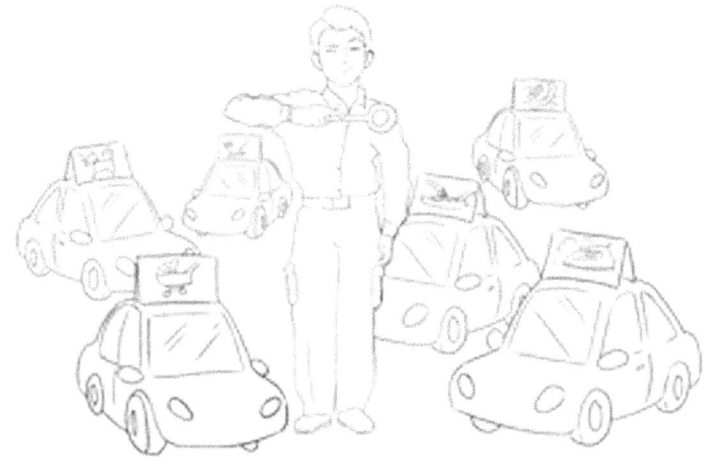

"À quoi penses-tu?"

(What are you thinking about?)

WOMEN CARRY INVISIBLE WEIGHTS

Dear Americans,

She remembers the Wi-Fi password, your cousin's allergy, the birthday gift for your mother, and which kid hates peas. You? You remember the TV remote. She carries an invisible backpack full of mental Post-its, and you wonder why she's tired. If you want her desire back, don't just bring flowers. Bring relief. Notice her effort. Share it. Take something off her shoulders before trying to take off her bra. Nothing is sexier than a woman who feels seen, supported, and free enough to want you.

Comme on dit en France:
Ce qu'elle porte ne se voit pas, mais ça l'épuise.

As we say in France:
What she carries can't be seen, but it drains her.

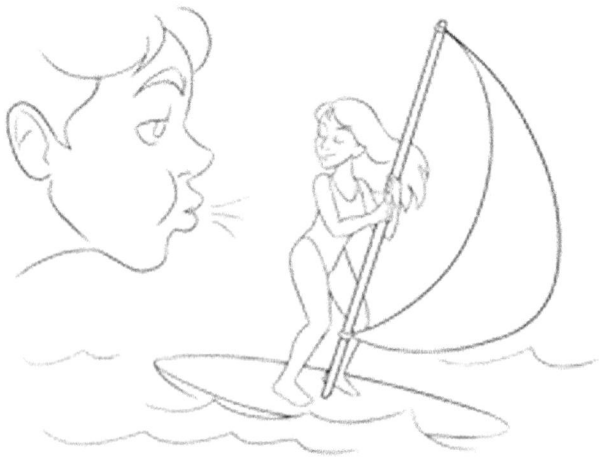

"À quoi penses-tu?"

(What are you thinking about?)

ANTICIPATION IS EROTIC

Dear Americans,

In France, we don't wait for instructions like interns on the first day of work. We notice. We anticipate. She sighs? We hear it. She looks tired. We act. Anticipation is not duty—it's seduction. Nothing is sexier than showing her you saw the need before she spoke it. Stop waiting for the PowerPoint presentation of "What Women Want." Desire begins with intuition, not permission slips. Be alert, be attuned—and suddenly, folding laundry becomes foreplay.

Comme on dit en France:
L'érotisme commence par l'intuition, pas l'instruction.

As we say in France:
Eroticism begins with intuition, not instruction.

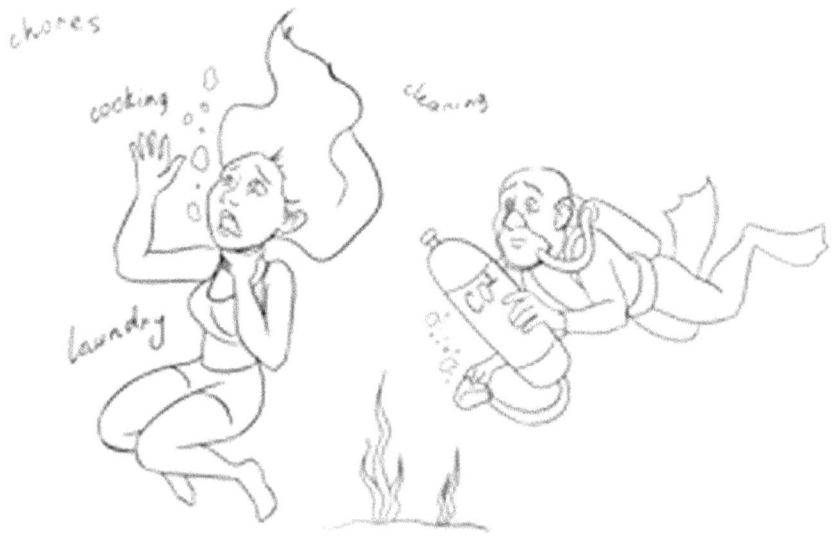

"À quoi penses-tu?"

(What are you thinking about?)

EMOTIONAL LABOR
IS PART OF FOREPLAY

Dear Americans,

You think foreplay starts with kissing? Non. It starts with the sentence: "What would make your day lighter?" instead of "What's for dinner?" Sexy, no? When her brain is carrying the weight of ten unpaid jobs, she's not fantasizing about lace, she's fantasizing about sleep. Ease her load, and you open the gates of desire. A relaxed mind is an aroused body. Forget roses; take out the trash. That's the French secret.

Comme on dit en France:
Soulager son esprit, c'est exciter son corps.

As we say in France:
Ease her mind, and you awaken her body.

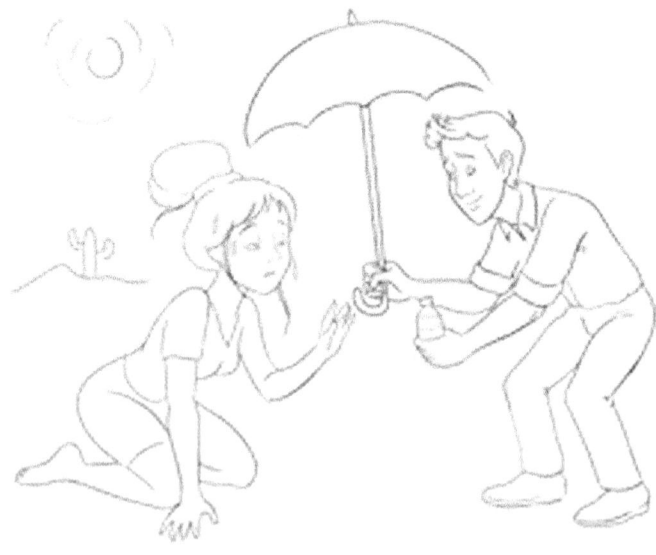

"À quoi penses-tu?"

(What are you thinking about?)

DON'T "HELP." LEAD.

Dear Americans,

Stop saying, "Tell me what to do." That's what interns say, not lovers. She doesn't need another assistant—she needs a partner. A man who notices, who acts, who doesn't need a gold star for running the dishwasher. Leadership in love is not domination; it's initiative. The sexiest thing you can do is fix the invisible without making a speech about it. Trust me, nothing kills desire faster than: "Look, honey, I put the plates away." Bravo... want a medal?

Comme on dit en France:
L'amour ne se prouve pas en demandant quoi faire,
mais en le faisant.

As we say in France:
Love isn't proven by asking what to do—but by doing it.

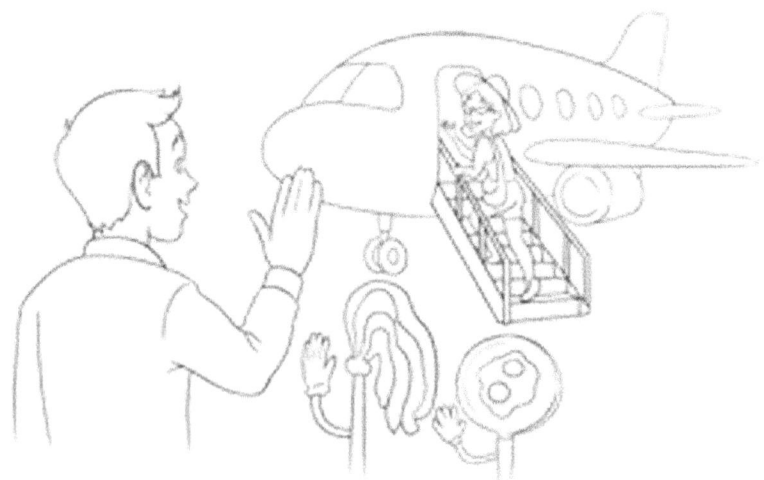

"À quoi penses-tu?"
(What are you thinking about?)

LOGISTICS CAN BE SEXY, TOO

Dear Americans,

You think seduction is roses, violins, champagne? Wrong. Sometimes it's handling the dentist appointment, ordering groceries, or booking the babysitter so she doesn't have to. Passion dies in exhaustion, but it comes alive in relief. You want her desire? Give her freedom from logistics. Plan the date—and not with a text that says, "So what do you wanna do?" Initiative is French foreplay. And let me tell you: Nothing turns her on like not being the household manager.

Comme on dit en France:
Le désir naît quand l'homme prend les devants.

As we say in France:
Desire is born when the man takes the lead.

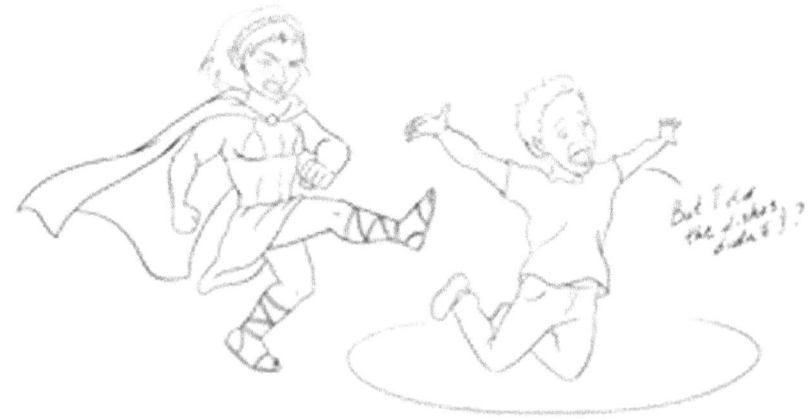

"À quoi penses-tu?"

(What are you thinking about?)

TAKE RESPONSIBILITY— NOT CREDIT

Dear Americans,

Doing dishes? Bathing kids? Cooking dinner? That's not foreplay, that's adulthood. Don't strut around waiting for applause like you just solved world hunger. "Look, honey, I vacuumed!" Bravo, mon héros. Here's your Nobel Prize in Domestic Affairs. No. A real man carries his share without turning it into theater. She doesn't need to clap; she needs to breathe. The sexiest thing isn't flowers—it's not having to mother her husband. Carry the load quietly, and she might carry you to bed.

Comme on dit en France:
Ce n'est pas une médaille, c'est ta mission.

As we say in France:
It's not a medal. It's your mission.

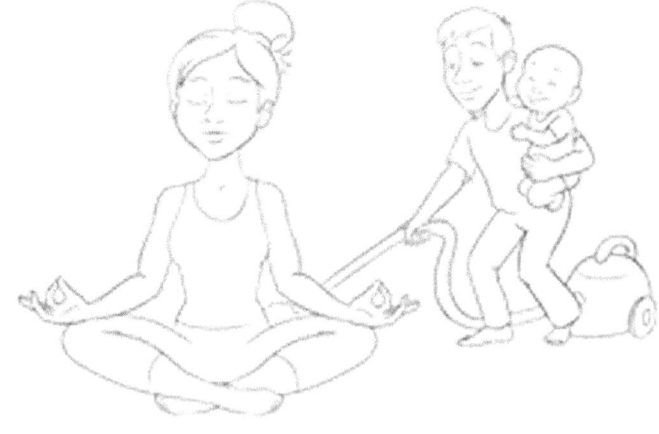

"À quoi penses-tu?"
(What are you thinking about?)

THE REAL BEDROOM BLOCKER ISN'T HER LIBIDO. IT'S HER LOAD.

Dear Americans,

She's not cold. She's not broken. She's simply fried. If she collapses into bed like a phone with 1 percent battery, it's not because she doesn't desire you; it's because she's been running on empty all day. Invisible lists, kids' chaos, bills—voilà, the libido killer. Passion doesn't die. It just hides under piles of laundry. If you want the heat back, don't buy lingerie— buy a mop. Share the weight, restore her energy, then watch her fire return.

Comme on dit en France:
Ce n'est pas son désir qui est mort, c'est son énergie qu'on a tuée.

As we say in France:
Her desire isn't dead. Her energy was killed.

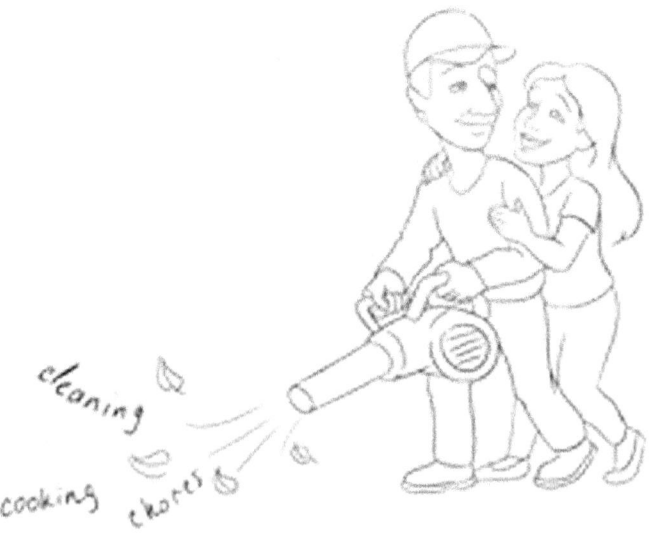

"À quoi penses-tu?"

(What are you thinking about?)

SHE DOESN'T WANT TO CARRY YOU

Dear Americans,

A woman doesn't want to feel like she's dragging a sack of potatoes through life. She wants a partner who can stand tall with her, not on her back. Love isn't one lonely pillar cracking under pressure while the other one scrolls through ESPN. Love is two columns, sharing the weight—and yes, sometimes the grocery bags, too. If she feels supported, she'll feel safe. And when she feels safe, she'll feel sexy. Strong shoulders aren't just for flexing; they're for lifting life together.

Comme on dit en France:
L'amour, c'est deux colonnes, pas une seule qui s'écroule.

As we say in France:
Love is two pillars, not one collapsing alone.

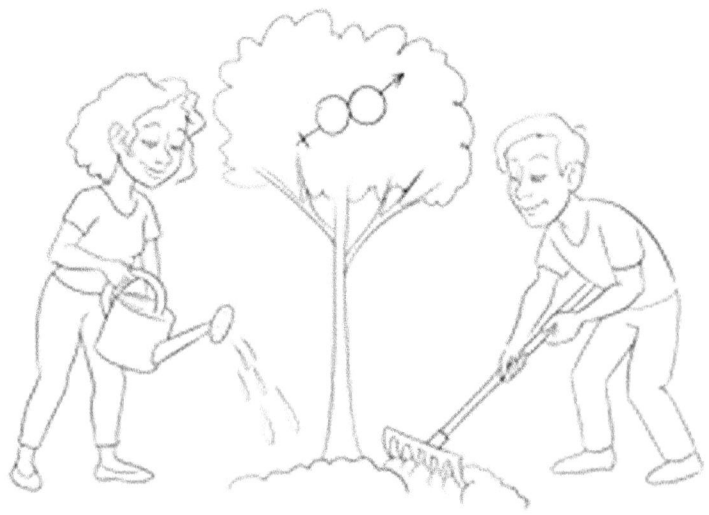

"À quoi penses-tu?"

(What are you thinking about?)

When She Feels Lighter, She Feels Sexier

Dear Americans,

Passion doesn't thrive in exhaustion; lust doesn't live in chaos. If she's juggling bills, kids, and dinner, she's not fantasizing about you—she's fantasizing about a nap. Liberation is foreplay. Take something off her plate, and suddenly she remembers she has a body, not just a to-do list. When her load lightens, her fire rises. It's not complicated: if you want her desire, start with the dishes. Voilà, sexiest dishwasher in town.

Comme on dit en France:
Soulager son quotidien, c'est réveiller son feu.

As we say in France:
Lighten her day, and you'll awaken her fire.

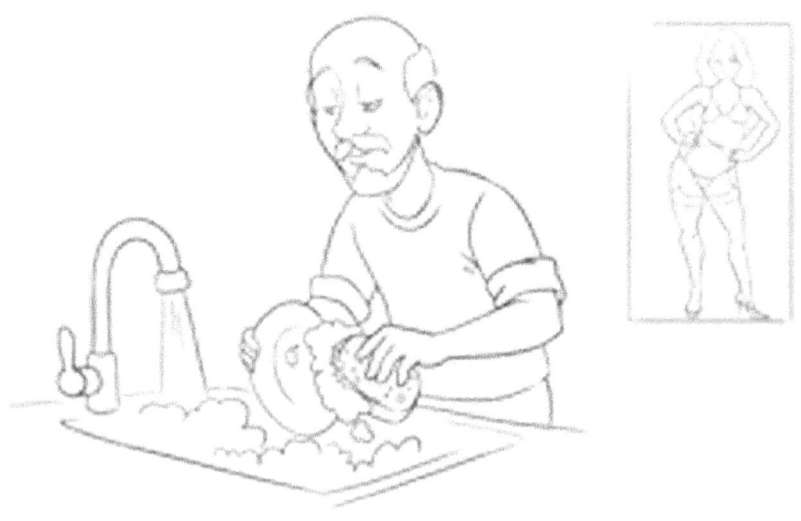

"À quoi penses-tu?"

(What are you thinking about?)

STOP EXPECTING HER TO WANT YOU WHEN SHE FEELS ALONE

Dear Americans,

Married loneliness doesn't always mean silence. Sometimes it's her carrying everything while you wonder why she isn't in the mood. If she's overworked, overstretched, and unseen, don't expect her to whisper, "Take me now." No, she's thinking, "Take this laundry instead." Passion cannot bloom in isolation. You want affection? Be her partner, not her spectator. Love is built on teamwork, and intimacy is the bonus prize.

Comme on dit en France:
Le désir ne fleurit pas dans la solitude du quotidien.

As we say in France:
Desire doesn't bloom in the loneliness of everyday life.

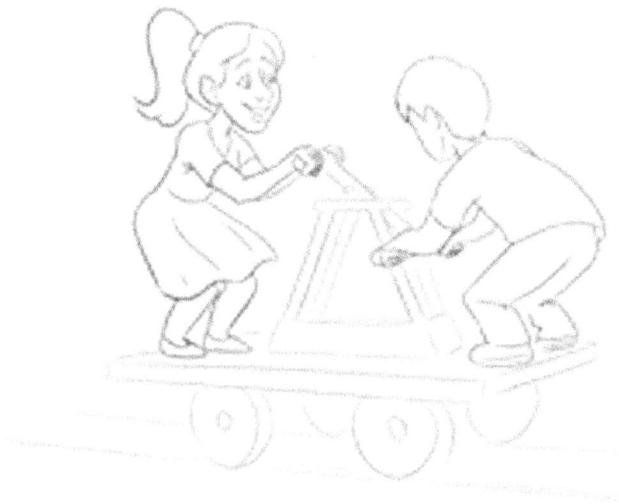

"À quoi penses-tu?"

(What are you thinking about?)

DESIRE IS A BYPRODUCT OF BALANCE

Dear Americans,

You can't manufacture desire with roses and reservations. You create it with balance. When she isn't drowning in responsibility, when laughter replaces resentment, when life feels lighter, her passion returns. Desire doesn't just disappear; it gets buried under imbalance. Help her find ease, and you'll find her longing again. Sexy isn't candlelight—it's vacuuming without being asked. Desire is not built. It's restored.

Comme on dit en France:
Le désir revient quand la vie redevient légère.

As we say in France:
Desire returns when life becomes light again.

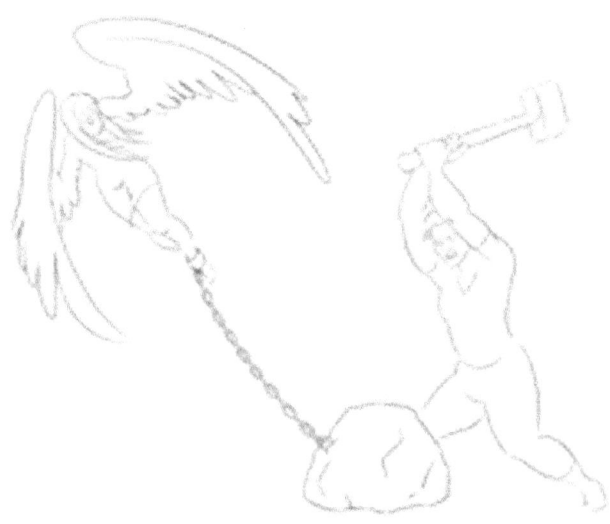

"À quoi penses-tu?"

(What are you thinking about?)

NOTHING IS COLDER THAN A MAN WHO'S PHYSICALLY THERE... BUT EMOTIONALLY GONE

Dear Americans,

There's nothing frostier than a man sitting on the couch while his soul is at the office, his eyes on the phone, and his brain inside ESPN highlights. She's not lonely because she's alone—she's lonely because you're there but absent. Every distracted "uh-huh" is a dagger. In France, we say a warm croissant is better than cold bread. Presence is the same: You can't reheat it later. If your heart is elsewhere, she knows.

Comme on dit en France:
Il est là, mais son cœur est ailleurs.

As we say in France:
He's there, but his heart is somewhere else.

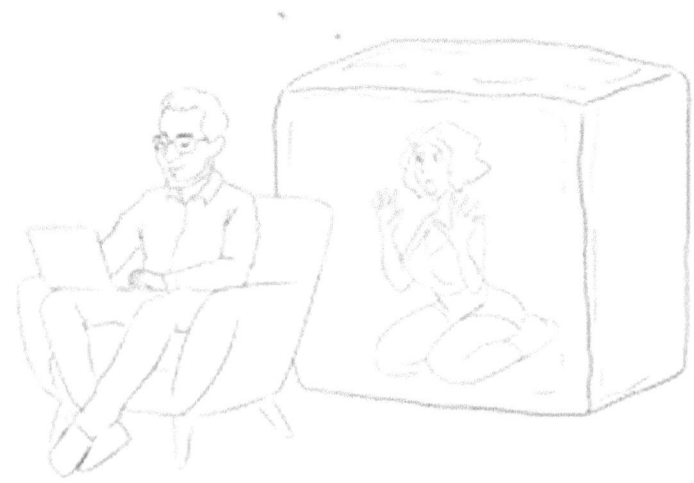

"À quoi penses-tu?"

(What are you thinking about?)

SILENCE CAN FEEL LIKE REJECTION

Dear Americans,

You think silence is safe. A little quiet can't hurt, right? Wrong. To her, silence isn't peace—it's rejection wearing pajamas. Every unsaid word screams louder than any argument. While you call it "neutral," she hears: "You don't matter." She'd rather fight, cry, or even throw a baguette at your head than face the vacuum of nothingness. In France, we argue loudly, kiss passionately, then eat cheese. Silence kills passion faster than any fight.

Comme on dit en France:
Le silence d'un homme crie plus fort qu'une dispute.

As we say in France:
A man's silence screams louder than a fight.

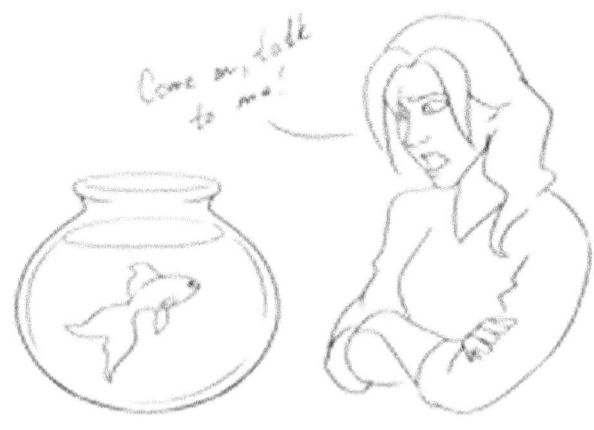

"À quoi penses-tu?"

(What are you thinking about?)

EMOTIONAL ABSENCE ISN'T SUBTLE. IT'S LOUD.

Dear Americans,

Men think that if they just keep quiet, nobody will notice the distance. Wrong again. Emotional absence makes more noise than a marching band. She feels it in shallow words, sees it in your drifting eyes, tastes it in your hollow kisses. You think you're hiding, but absence rings like a fire alarm in the soul. In France, we know that wine without flavor tastes like betrayal. Emotional absence? It's worse than an argument. At least fights prove you're alive.

Comme on dit en France:
L'absence émotionnelle, ça s'entend même dans le silence.

As we say in France:
Emotional absence is heard even in silence.

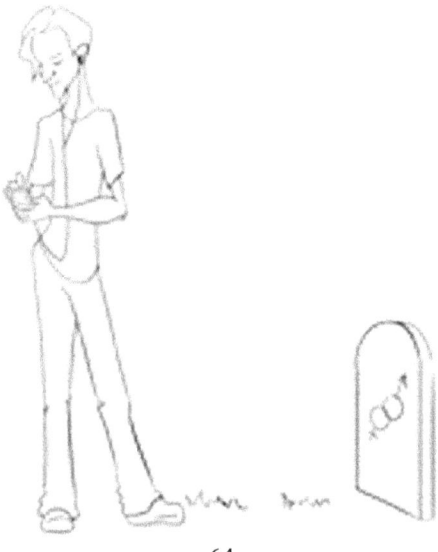

"À quoi penses-tu?"

(What are you thinking about?)

SHE DOESN'T WANT YOU TO FIX IT. SHE WANTS YOU TO FEEL IT WITH HER.

Dear Americans,

She doesn't need another handyman. She needs a human. When she shares pain, stop reaching for duct tape solutions. She's not broken—she's burdened. Sit. Listen. Breathe with her. Don't manage her feelings like you manage a calendar. Presence is not about fixing; it's about witnessing. In France, we know sometimes the most romantic act is simply holding silence together with empathy. Stop fixing the plumbing of her heart. Just sit inside it with her. That's intimacy.

Comme on dit en France:
Le cœur n'a pas besoin de solutions, juste d'un témoin.

As we say in France:
The heart doesn't need fixing—just a witness.

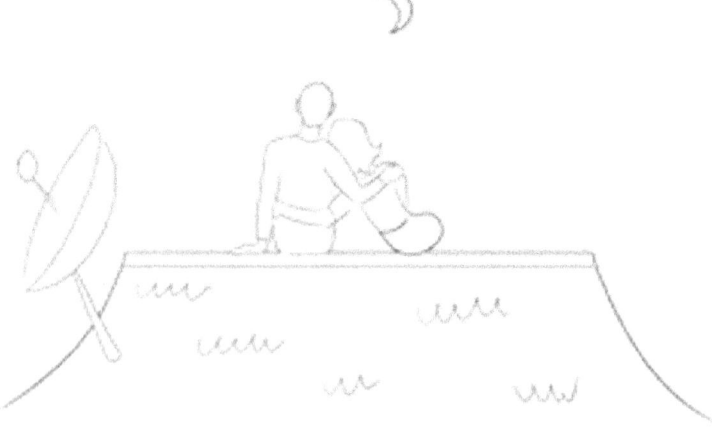

"À quoi penses-tu?"

(What are you thinking about?)

TOUCH WITHOUT PRESENCE IS JUST CONTACT

Dear Americans,

Anyone can touch. Few can connect. She feels the difference between hands that grope like they're punching a time clock, and hands that linger like they've discovered treasure. Touch without presence is paperwork. Touch with presence is poetry. You can't fake it. Even with her eyes closed, she knows if your soul is absent. In France, we say a kiss without passion is just lip cardio. Don't give her cardio—give her communion. That's when touch becomes timeless.

Comme on dit en France:
La présence se sent, même les yeux fermés.

As we say in France:
Presence is felt—even with eyes closed.

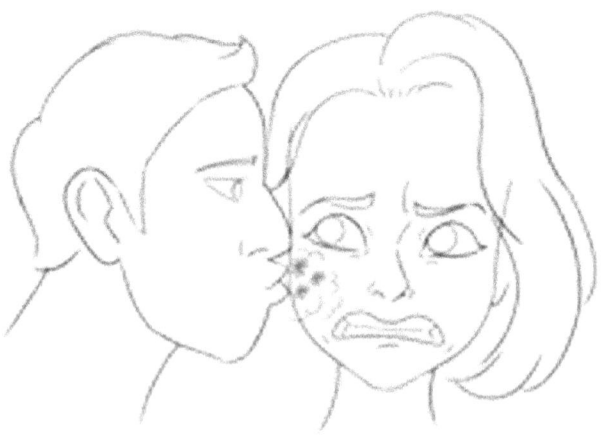

68

"À quoi penses-tu?"
(What are you thinking about?)

REPLACE "WHAT'S FOR DINNER?" WITH "WHAT'S ON YOUR MIND?"

Dear Americans,

Asking "What's for dinner?" is not intimacy; it's laziness with seasoning. Try asking her: "What's weighing on your mind?" or "What dream are you hiding?" Trust me, pasta won't seduce her, but curiosity will. Connection begins in the soul, not the shopping list. In France, we feed the mind first, then the stomach—and both end up satisfied. Dinner can wait, but her heart cannot.

Comme on dit en France:
La vraie faim, c'est d'être compris.

As we say in France:
The real hunger is to be understood.

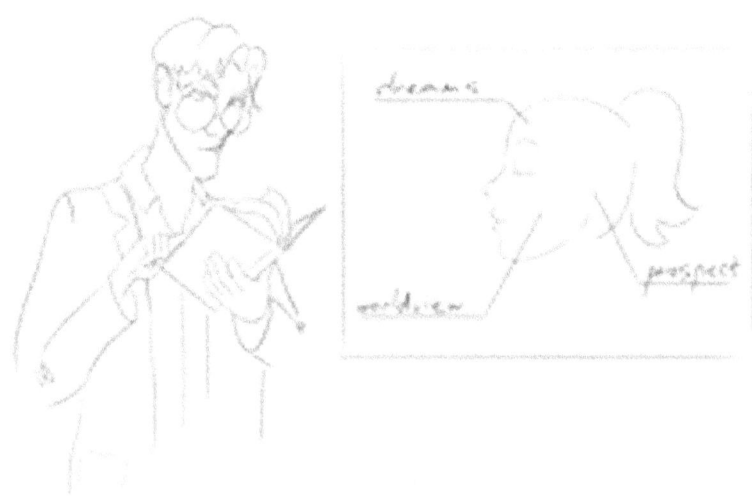

"À quoi penses-tu?"
(What are you thinking about?)

SHE DOESN'T WANT YOUR PERFECTION. SHE WANTS YOUR EMOTION.

Dear Americans,

Perfection is for résumés. Emotion is for romance. Hiding behind "I'm fine" makes you sound like a malfunctioning robot. She doesn't need the polished, LinkedIn version of you. She wants the raw, unfiltered you who admits fear, joy, longing. Cry if you must. Laugh awkwardly. Be messy. In France, we know wine tastes better with flaws than with fakery. Authenticity is the fire; perfection is the extinguisher.

Comme on dit en France:
L'amour vrai ne porte pas de masque.

As we say in France:
True love wears no mask.

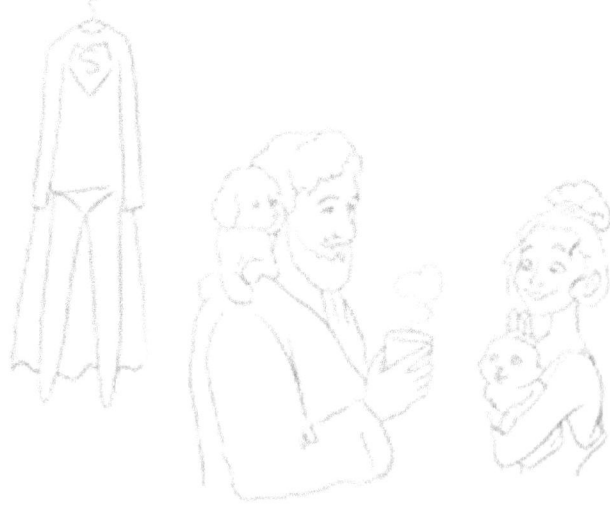

"À quoi penses-tu?"
(What are you thinking about?)

PHYSICAL PRESENCE ISN'T EMOTIONAL PRESENCE

Dear Americans,

Sleeping in the same bed doesn't mean you're present. Dogs sleep in beds, too. What she craves isn't just your body heat but your heart heat. If your mind is wandering through emails while you lie next to her, you're basically a space heater. In France, we know proximity is geography; intimacy is depth. Don't just be there. Arrive. Entirely.

Comme on dit en France:
Être là, ce n'est pas être présent.

As we say in France:
Being there isn't the same as being present.

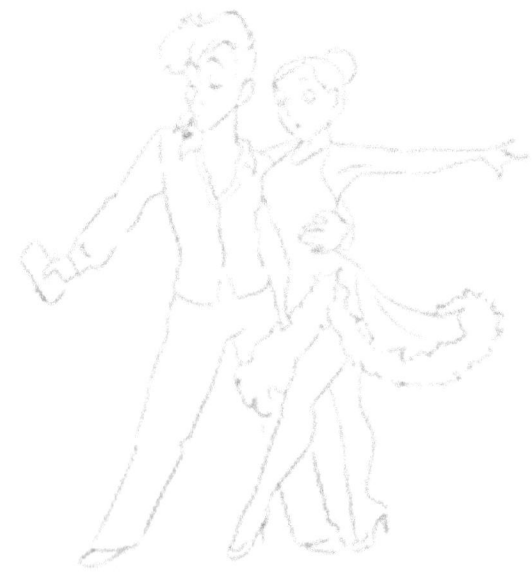

"À quoi penses-tu?"
(What are you thinking about?)

DON'T WAIT FOR HER TO BEG FOR CONNECTION

Dear Americans,

If she has to whisper, "I feel alone beside you," then mon ami, you've already lost the plot. Don't wait for her to file a complaint with HR. Anticipate before despair sets in. In France, we don't let bread go stale on the counter. Why would you let love do the same? Lean in before she pulls away. Connection is a gift, not a negotiation.

Comme on dit en France:
L'absence se sent, même à deux centimètres.

As we say in France:
Absence can be felt—even from two inches away.

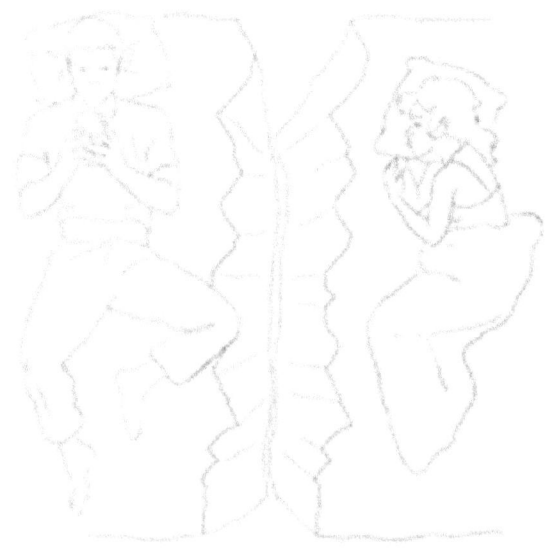

"À quoi penses-tu?"

(What are you thinking about?)

DESIRE STARTS WITH ATTENTION, NOT TECHNIQUE

Dear Americans,

You think technique is everything—speed, rhythm, tricks. But without attention, it's just gymnastics. Look into your partner's eyes, not to "ask permission," but to see. That sincere gaze is the green light passion runs on. Forget tequila shots and cheesy pick-up lines; presence is the aphrodisiac. In France, we know one sincere look can melt more clothes than a thousand moves.

Comme on dit en France:
Un regard sincère vaut mille caresses.

As we say in France:
One sincere gaze is worth a thousand caresses.

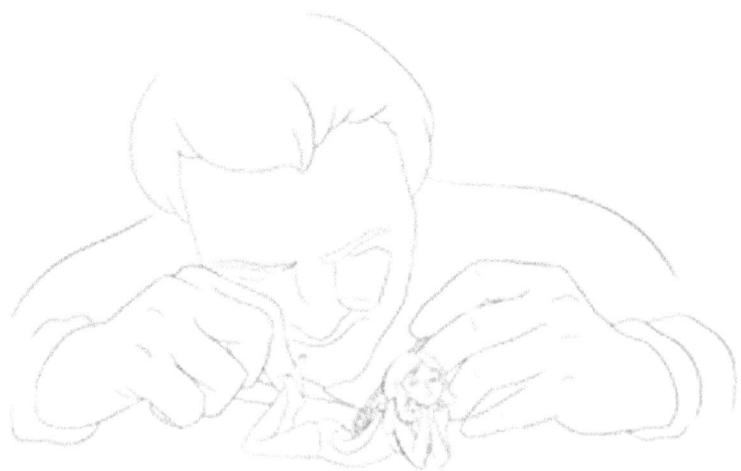

"À quoi penses-tu?"

(What are you thinking about?)

THE FRENCH MAN'S FOREPLAY DOESN'T START IN BED

Dear Americans,

Foreplay doesn't begin at midnight—it begins at 6 p.m. with a kiss in the kitchen or a hand brushing her shoulder. Massage is not pressure; it's painting. Don't rush like an athlete chasing trophies. Stroke like an artist, awakening colors. Desire is not pushed; it simmers. That's why French cuisine and French love share the same secret: slow heat.

Comme on dit en France:
Le désir se peint, il ne se pousse pas.

As we say in France:
Desire is painted, not pushed.

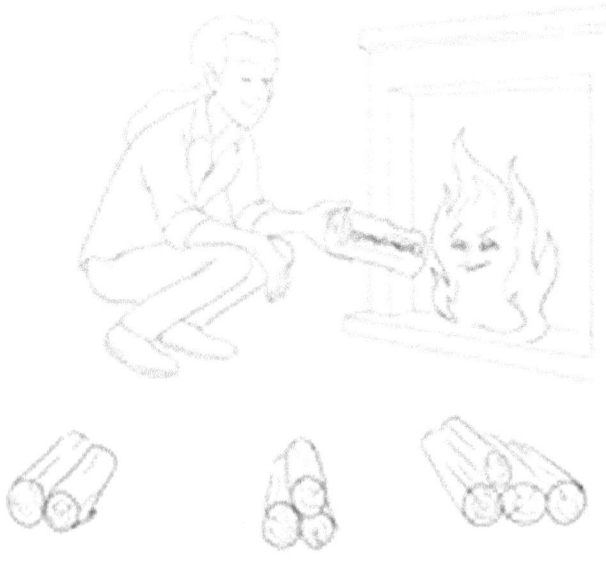

"À quoi penses-tu?"
(What are you thinking about?)

KISSING ISN'T A STEP. IT'S A LANGUAGE.

Dear Americans,

A kiss is not a checkpoint—it's a whole dialogue. In France, we know lips are storytellers. A teasing kiss says, "wait for it." A deep one says, "I'm lost." A playful brush whispers, "I cherish you." Too many men treat kissing like the trailer instead of the movie. Wrong. Master her mouth, and you master her heart. Skip it, and you'll never reach her soul. A kiss is not foreplay—it's poetry.

Comme on dit en France:
Un baiser est un poème sans mots.

As we say in France:
A kiss is a poem without words.

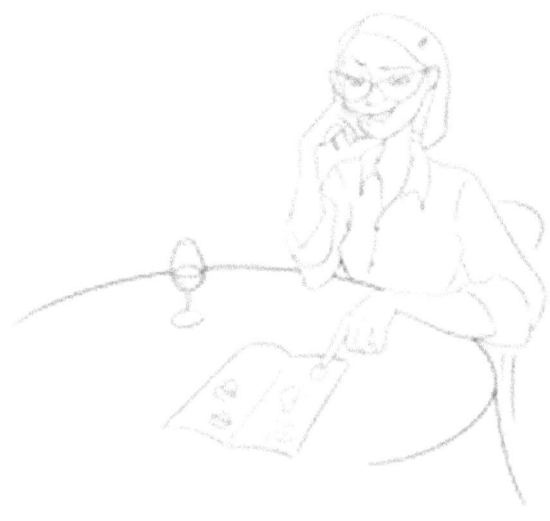

"À quoi penses-tu?"

(What are you thinking about?)

WORSHIP, DON'T RUSH

Dear Americans,

Her breasts are not pit stops on the way to "the main event." They are sacred monuments—cathedrals, not checkpoints. Don't grope—worship. Touch them as though you were reading Braille in the dark, searching for a secret. Linger. Kiss. Play. A woman who feels revered in your mouth will surrender her entire body. Worship transforms lust into intimacy, and intimacy into devotion. Men who rush are amateurs. Men who worship? They are unforgettable.

Comme on dit en France:
Le corps d'une femme est une cathédrale.

As we say in France:
A woman's body is a cathedral.

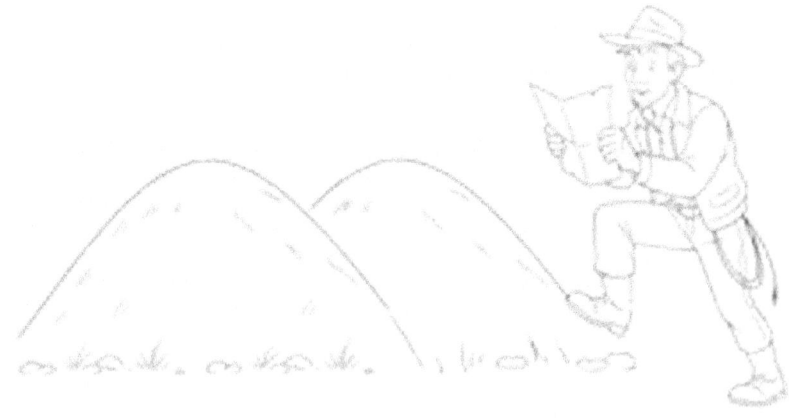

"À quoi penses-tu?"

(What are you thinking about?)

THERE ARE TWO KINGDOMS— CLITORAL AND VAGINAL

Dear Americans,

Women are not universal remotes with one button. Some melt with rhythm, others with depth. Some need clitoral devotion, others the embrace of penetration. The trick? Listen. Not with your ears but with your hands, lips, eyes. Her body speaks: the arch of her back, the tremor in her voice, the rise of her hips. Don't force your manual—read hers. Every woman has her own key. If you're smart, you'll learn the lock.

Comme on dit en France:
Chaque femme a sa clé. Apprends sa serrure.

As we say in France:
Every woman has her key. Learn her lock.

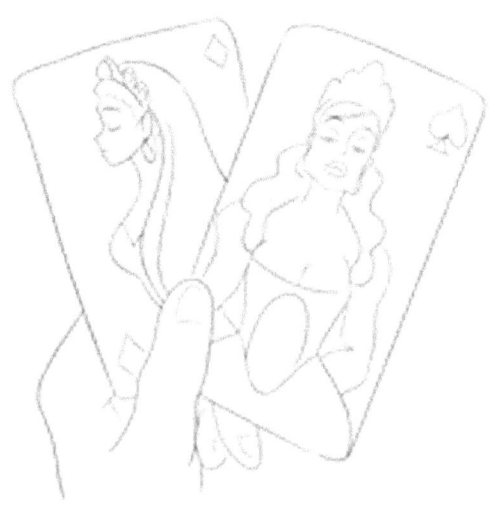

"À quoi penses-tu?"

(What are you thinking about?)

SEND HER TO HEAVEN.
THEN RETURN TO EARTH.

Dear Americans,

Too many men climax like sprinters and collapse like corpses. Amateur hour. In France, we know ecstasy is the beginning of romance, not the end. After the fireworks, kiss her again. Hold her. Trace her skin like you're signing a love letter. Let her know she's still the center, not the sideshow. Orgasms fade. Connection stays. If you want her tomorrow, romance her after today.

Comme on dit en France:
L'extase n'est que le début du câlin.

As we say in France:
Ecstasy is only the beginning of the embrace.

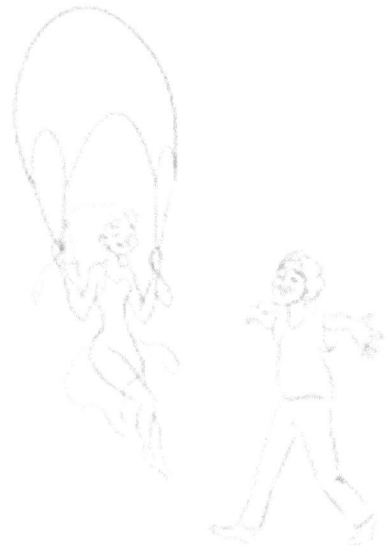

"À quoi penses-tu?"

(What are you thinking about?)

IT'S NOT ABOUT POSITIONS. IT'S ABOUT INTENTION.

Dear Americans,

Missionary can be divine. Cowgirl can be liberating. Doggy can be wild instinct. None of it matters if your mind is elsewhere. Passion isn't created by angles—it's created by attention. You can fold her into a thousand poses, but if you're absent, it's just gymnastics. Desire isn't about how you bend; it's about how you show up. Presence, not position, is what makes her shiver.

Comme on dit en France:
Ce n'est pas la pose, c'est la présence.

As we say in France:
It's not the position—it's the presence.

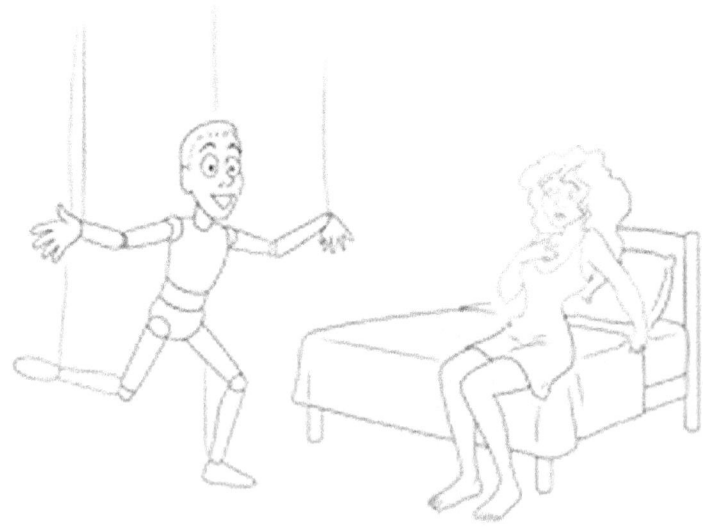

"À quoi penses-tu?"

(What are you thinking about?)

PROTECTION ISN'T JUST PHYSICAL. IT'S RESPECTFUL.

Dear Americans,

A condom doesn't kill desire—carelessness does. True seduction is safety wrapped in passion. When you protect her body, you protect her trust. And trust is the true aphrodisiac. She wants a lover who cares not only for the night but for tomorrow. Respect is sexy. Responsibility is seductive. Any man can be reckless. A real man knows devotion requires protection.

Comme on dit en France:
La sécurité peut aussi être sexy.

As we say in France:
Safety can also be sexy.

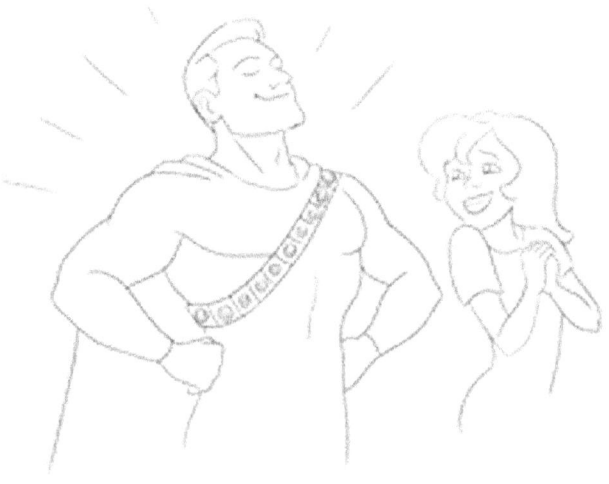

"À quoi penses-tu?"

(What are you thinking about?)

DON'T PERFORM. CONNECT.

Dear Americans,

Stop turning the bedroom into a CrossFit class. It's not about reps, speed, or stamina. This isn't theater—it's intimacy. She doesn't want a showman; she wants a partner who listens with his hands and responds with his soul. Connection beats duration every single time. When her pleasure becomes yours, orgasm stops being a finish line—it becomes a shared dialogue. Forget the stopwatch. Learn her breath.

Comme on dit en France:
L'orgasme est un dialogue, pas un spectacle.

As we say in France:
Orgasm is a dialogue, not a performance.

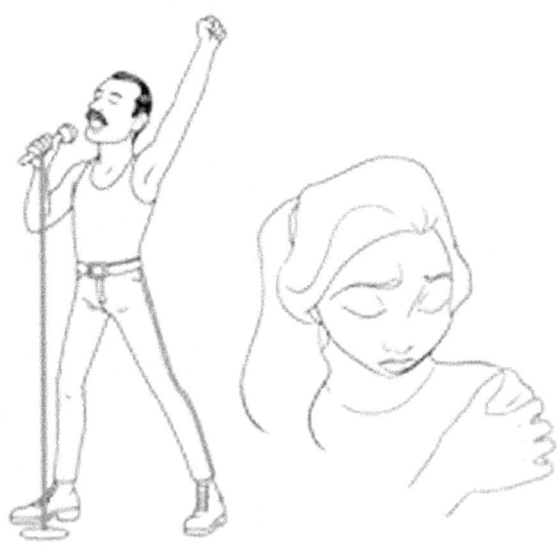

"À quoi penses-tu?"

(What are you thinking about?)

IF HER BODY SINGS, DON'T CHANGE THE SONG

Dear Americans,

Nothing kills the symphony faster than a DJ boyfriend. She's moaning, arching, trembling—her whole body screaming "Encore!" And what do you do? Switch the track. Change the beat. Try a trick you saw online. Stop. If her body is singing under your rhythm, stay in the music. Consistency is mastery, not confusion. In France, we don't remix what already melts her—we repeat it until she dissolves completely.

Comme on dit en France:
Ne change pas une recette qui fait fondre.

As we say in France:
Don't change a recipe that melts hearts.

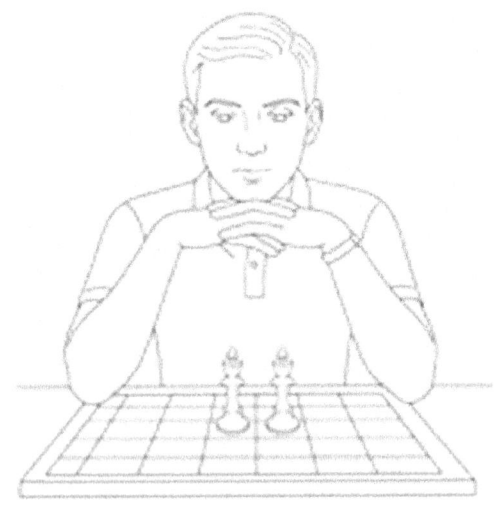

"À quoi penses-tu?"

(What are you thinking about?)

SLOW DOWN.
THEN SLOW DOWN AGAIN.

Dear Americans,

Speed is for Wi-Fi, not women. Too many of you rush like you're trying to catch a train. Desire thrives in suspense, not shortcuts. Let your fingers wander. Let your tongue linger. Stretch the silence until it aches with anticipation. Every pause builds hunger; every delay makes the climax volcanic. If you rush, you'll have sex. If you slow down, you'll have seduction. And seduction, my friends, is what she'll remember.

Comme on dit en France:
Plus tu attends, plus c'est bon.

As we say in France:
The longer you wait, the better it gets.

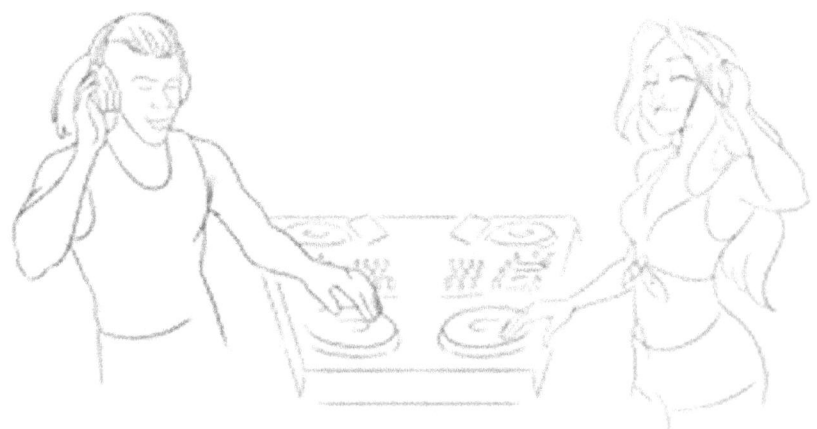

"À quoi penses-tu?"

(What are you thinking about?)

TALK LESS. FEEL MORE.

Dear Americans,

You're not sports commentators, so stop narrating every move. "Do you like this? How about this?" Non. Her body is already speaking—through her breath, her thighs, her sighs. Listen with your hands. Learn with your lips. In France, real lovers know silence can be sexier than a thousand dirty words. Words may flatter, but presence ignites. Trust her body to tell you where to go. Trust yourself to hear it. That's when intimacy stops being mechanical—and becomes instinct.

Comme on dit en France:
Quand les lèvres se taisent, les mains deviennent éloquentes.

As we say in France:
When lips fall silent, the hands become eloquent.

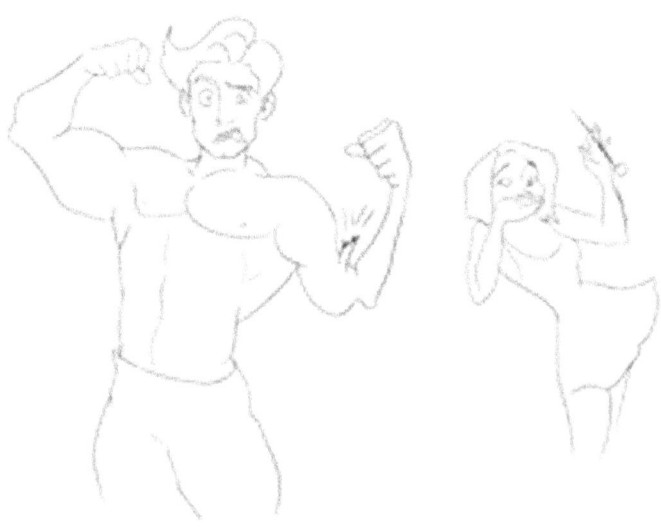

"À quoi penses-tu?"
(What are you thinking about?)

TRUTH #51

AFTER YOU TAKE HER TO HEAVEN, DON'T VANISH

Dear Americans,

Too many men climax like fireworks and disappear like smoke. But in France, we know the afterglow is sacred. When she melts, don't roll away—roll closer. Kiss her. Hold her. Trace lazy circles down her back. Remind her she wasn't just a performance, but your partner. Orgasms fade, but tenderness lingers. The memory she keeps is not the explosion, but the embrace that follows. And that's where love grows again.

Comme on dit en France:
L'extase finit dans les bras, pas sur le côté.

As we say in France:
Ecstasy ends in the arms, not on the side of the bed.

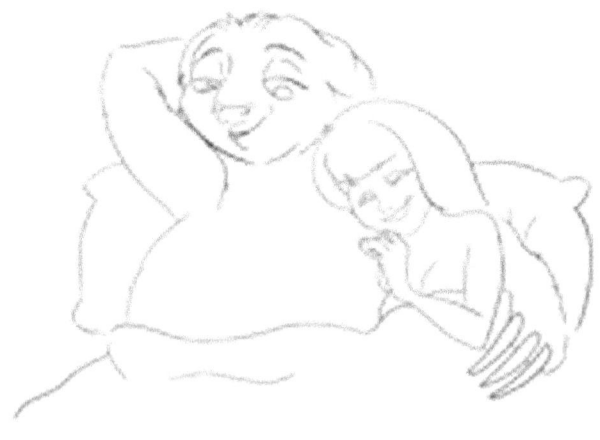

"À quoi penses-tu?"

(What are you thinking about?)

SHE'S NOT A SWITCH. YOU CAN'T JUST TURN HER ON.

Dear Americans,

Your wife isn't Alexa or Siri—you can't shout "Turn on!" at midnight and expect fireworks. Desire doesn't flick on like a lamp; it builds like a slow flame. She needs warmth, anticipation, laughter. It starts with a look at breakfast, a cheeky text at lunch, a playful touch in the hallway. By bedtime, she's already lit. In France, we know a match burns brighter if you caress it first. Treat her with the same patience. Don't flip her switch—stoke her fire.

Comme on dit en France:
Une allumette brûle mieux quand elle est caressée.

As we say in France:
A match burns better when it's gently stroked.

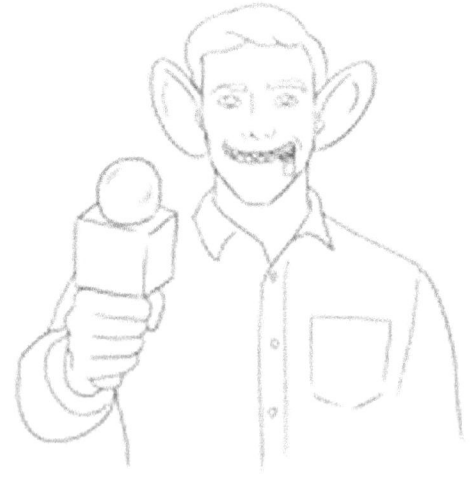

"À quoi penses-tu?"
(What are you thinking about?)

HER PLEASURE IS YOUR PASSPORT

Dear Americans,

Penetration isn't a passport stamp. Her pleasure is. If her toes curl, if her back arches, if your name escapes like a prayer—you've arrived. In France, we say that if she doesn't climax, you didn't finish the meal. Because sex isn't fast food—it's fine dining. You must taste, savor, and simmer. A woman isn't conquered by ego; she surrenders to devotion. Cook her pleasure carefully, and she'll serve you fire. Forget conquest—her bliss is the only stamp that counts.

Comme on dit en France:
Sa jouissance, c'est ton passeport.

As we say in France:
Her climax is your passport.

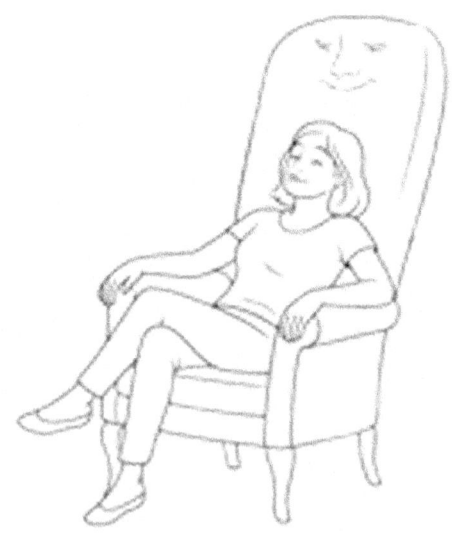

106

"À quoi penses-tu?"

(What are you thinking about?)

ONE POSITION DOESN'T FIT ALL

Dear Americans,

Missionary position can be poetry. Cowgirl can be freedom. Doggy can be wildfire. But the Kama Sutra won't save you if you're absent. Too many chase acrobatics instead of atmosphere. In France, we laugh at this circus. Desire isn't about geometry—it's about intention. Make her feel safe, seen, wanted, and even the simplest touch becomes symphony. Don't collect positions like baseball cards. Collect moments. That's how passion lives.

Comme on dit en France:
L'amour n'a pas de posture, seulement des intentions.

As we say in France:
Love has no pose—only intention.

Loading

"À quoi penses-tu?"

(What are you thinking about?)

EYE CONTACT
ISN'T JUST FOR THE FIRST DATE

Dear Americans,

Why do you close your eyes during sex—are you shy, or rehearsing lines? In France, we know the eyes are part of foreplay. One glance can melt resistance; one smirk can ignite fire. Look at her—not in a creepy, interrogation way—but in a "I see you, I'm with you" way. Eyes say what lips can't: presence. Soul. Intimacy. Lovers who never break eye contact don't just make love to the body. They seduce the spirit. That's erotic. That's unforgettable.

Comme on dit en France:
Un regard vrai deshabille plus qu'une main.

As we say in France:
A true gaze undresses more than a hand.

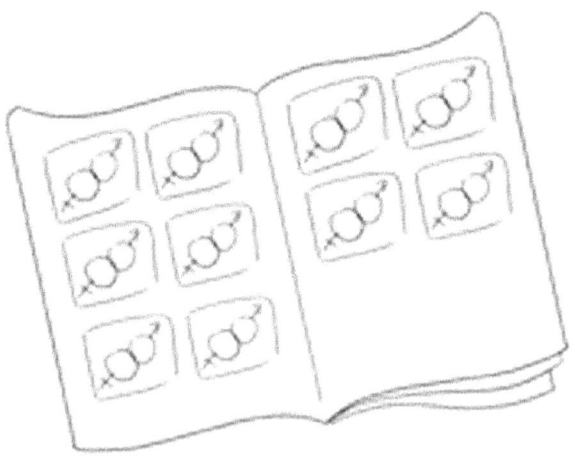

"À quoi penses-tu?"

(What are you thinking about?)

YOUR HANDS SHOULD LEARN HER LIKE BRAILLE

Dear Americans,

Stop groping like you're fumbling for the TV remote. Her body is not a puzzle to solve. It's a novel to read. Every scar, curve, and shiver is a paragraph. Touch her shoulder like it hides a secret. Trace her hip like it's art. Glide across her skin as though you're deciphering poetry. French lovers don't "grab"—we listen with our palms. Each caress is a sentence. Each pause is punctuation. Read her slowly, and you'll discover entire libraries of pleasure.

Comme on dit en France:
Chaque femme est un poème qu'on lit avec la peau.

As we say in France:
Every woman is a poem you read with your skin.

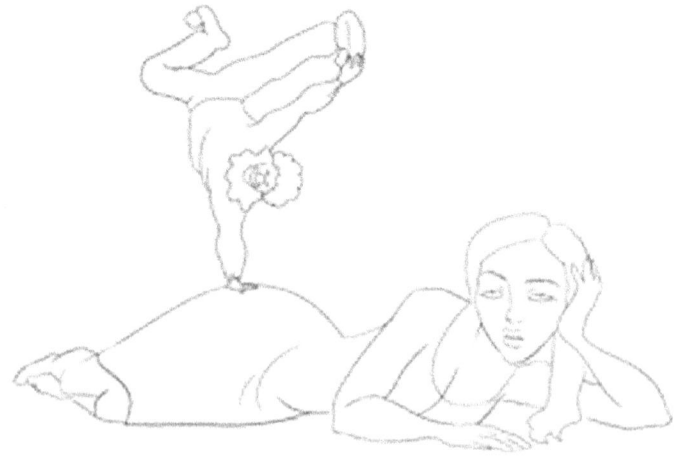

"À quoi penses-tu?"

(What are you thinking about?)

IF YOU'RE SILENT, SHE MIGHT THINK YOU'RE ABSENT

Dear Americans,

Silence can be romantic—on a walk by the river, not in bed. In the sheets, silence feels like absence. She doesn't need a TED Talk, but she does need proof you're there. A whisper: "You're beautiful." A moan: "You taste like heaven." A sign that says: "I'm lost in you." That's the connection. In France, moans are music, not mistakes. Whispers are poetry, not performance. One careless silence feels like rejection; one tender word can undo walls. Choose words. They linger longer than thrusts.

Comme on dit en France:
Un homme muet au lit, c'est un fantôme avec des draps.

As we say in France:
A silent man in bed is just a ghost with sheets.

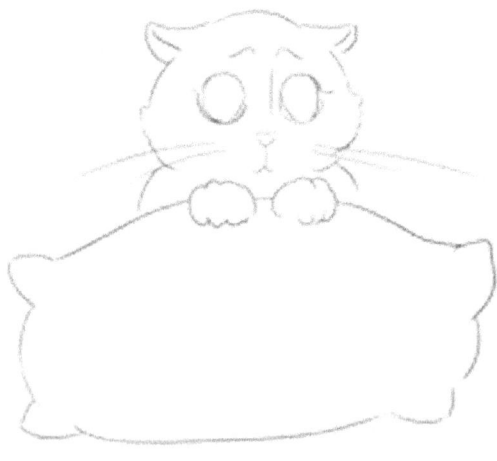

"À quoi penses-tu?"

(What are you thinking about?)

DON'T ASK IF SHE CAME—FEEL IT

Dear Americans,

If you must ask, you weren't there. Her back arches, her hips shudder, her breath catches—her body is practically yelling the answer. Yet you whisper, "Did you come?" as if it's a customer survey. French men know: The best chefs don't check the clock. They taste, they sense, they know when the dish is ready. Your lover is the same. Learn her recipe. Stay in her rhythm. Don't tick boxes. Feel the storm. That's the difference between clueless and connected.

Comme on dit en France:
Les meilleurs chefs savent quand le plat est prêt, sans minuteur.

As we say in France:
The best chefs know when the dish is ready—no timer needed.

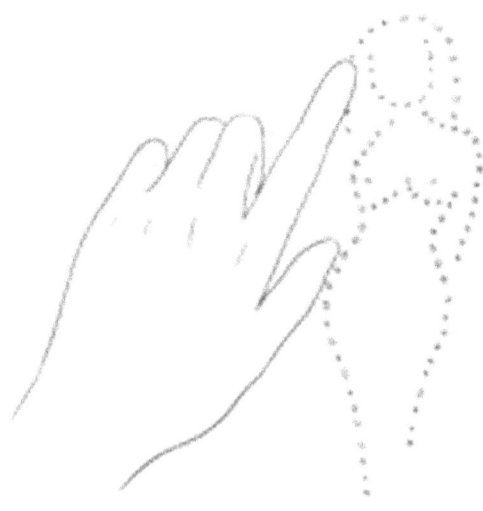

"À quoi penses-tu?"
(What are you thinking about?)

THE AFTERGLOW IS WHERE LOVE GROWS

Dear Americans,

Stop rolling over like you just finished a CrossFit set. The orgasm isn't the finale—it's the opening credits of tenderness. Hold her. Kiss her forehead. Trace her lips like you're sketching art. Let her know she was more than release—she was communion. In France, we treat the afterglow as sacred. It's where silence becomes poetry, where bodies rest but hearts dance. If you grab your phone, you've killed the mood. If you linger, you've built devotion.

Comme on dit en France:
L'amour continue dans les silences, pas seulement dans les soupirs.

As we say in France:
Love continues in the silences, not just in the sighs.

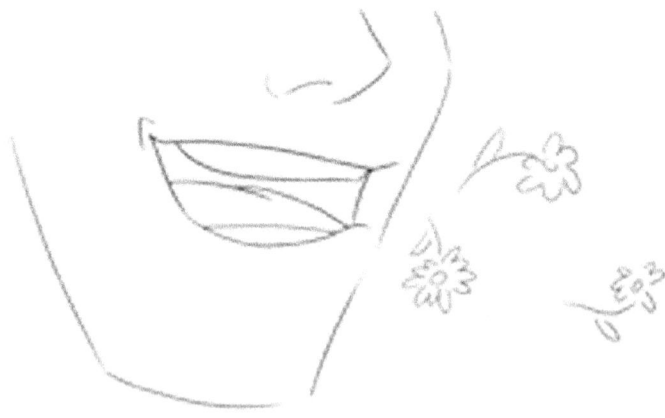

"À quoi penses-tu?"

(What are you thinking about?)

DON'T JUST UNDRESS HER. REVEAL HER.

Dear Americans,

Any fool can rip off a blouse. But only a lover knows how to peel away the armor she wears from stress, doubts, responsibilities. Undress slowly, with reverence. Each button undone should whisper: "I see you. I choose you." Don't strip her like luggage at TSA. Treat her like an unopened bottle of Bordeaux—with patience, ritual, anticipation. In France, we know undressing is not conquest; it's ceremony. Reveal her essence, not just her skin.

Comme on dit en France:
Si tu ouvres une femme comme une valise,
ne t'étonne pas qu'elle reste fermée.

As we say in France:
If you open a woman like luggage,
don't be surprised if she stays closed.

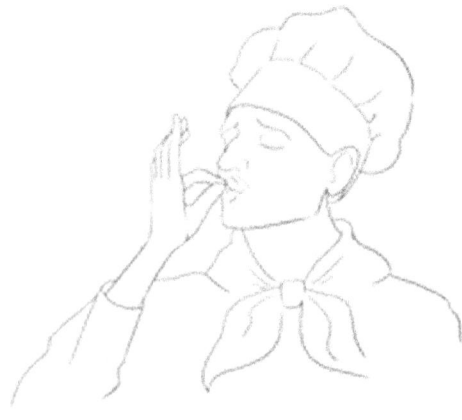

"À quoi penses-tu?"

(What are you thinking about?)

IF YOU WANT HER WILD, MAKE HER FEEL SAFE FIRST

Dear Americans,

You can't demand that she unleash her wild side while you make her feel judged, rushed, or dismissed. A caged heart never roars. But when she feels safe, adored, protected? She transforms into fire with oxygen. Tenderness is the doorway to her rawest passion. Hold her like you'll never drop her, and she'll give you what no performance could. French men know safety isn't boring—it's the sexiest foundation for freedom.

Comme on dit en France:
La sécurité émotionnelle est l'oreiller du plaisir.

As we say in France:
Emotional safety is the pillow of pleasure.

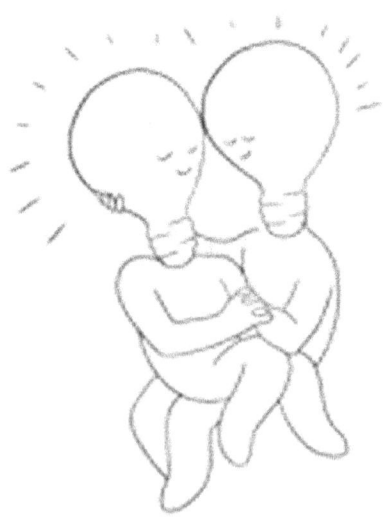

"À quoi penses-tu?"
(What are you thinking about?)

DON'T IMITATE PORN.
INSPIRE INTIMACY.

Dear Americans,

Porn is fiction—edited lighting, fake moans, scripted angles. If you're copying Pornhub choreography, you're not making love, you're auditioning. She doesn't want a star. She wants a partner. Kiss because you crave her, not because you saw it in a thumbnail. Touch because you feel her, not because it looked hot on mute. French men don't rehearse—we improvise. Real intimacy is messy, funny, and beautiful. Don't perform. Connect. That's sex worth remembering.

Comme on dit en France:
Si tu veux du cinéma, va au cinéma. Au lit, on veut du vrai.

As we say in France:
If you want cinema, go to the movies. In bed, we want the real thing.

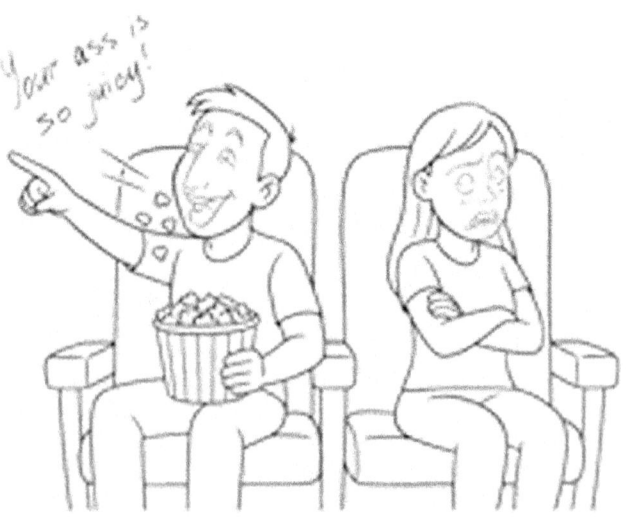

"À quoi penses-tu?"

(What are you thinking about?)

SHE DOESN'T WANT YOU PERFECT. SHE WANTS YOU PRESENT.

Dear Americans,

You'll bump noses. Lose rhythm. Maybe even fall off the bed. So what? She's not auditioning you for Cirque du Soleil. She doesn't need a flawless actor. She wants a present partner. Notice her breath. Pause when she tenses. Laugh when it's clumsy. Perfection is sterile; presence is sexy. French lovers know tenderness forgives everything. And the ability to stay with her—not above her, not apart from her—is what makes intimacy unforgettable.

Comme on dit en France:
La tendresse rattrape tout.

As we say in France:
Tenderness makes up for everything.

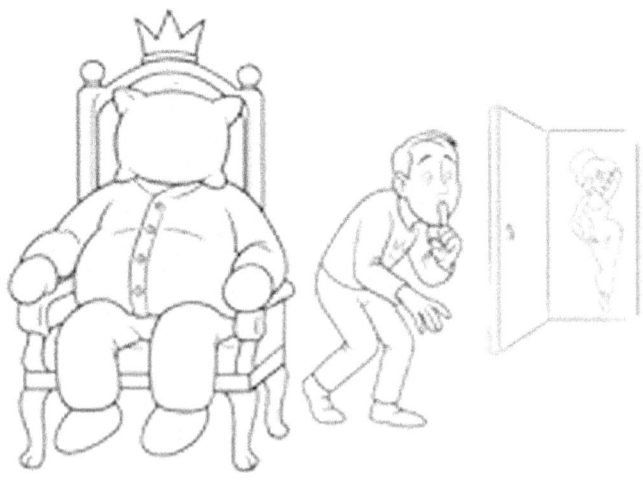

"À quoi penses-tu?"

(What are you thinking about?)

CONFIDENCE IS SEXY. CONSENT IS SEXIER

Dear Americans,

Confidence excites. It makes her body lean in. But push too far, and she'll retreat faster than a cat near water. Real seduction isn't force—it's presence. Lead with boldness, yes, but lace it with respect. Consent isn't a mood killer; it's the very oxygen of passion. In France, we don't steal kisses; we stage them, so they're freely given. Confidence without consent is arrogance. Consent with confidence. That's irresistible. True seduction is making her feel wanted and safe in the same breath. That's not weakness—it's mastery.

Comme on dit en France:
Le non est une porte fermée, mais le oui… c'est Versailles.

As we say in France:
"No" is a closed door, but "Yes"… that's Versailles.

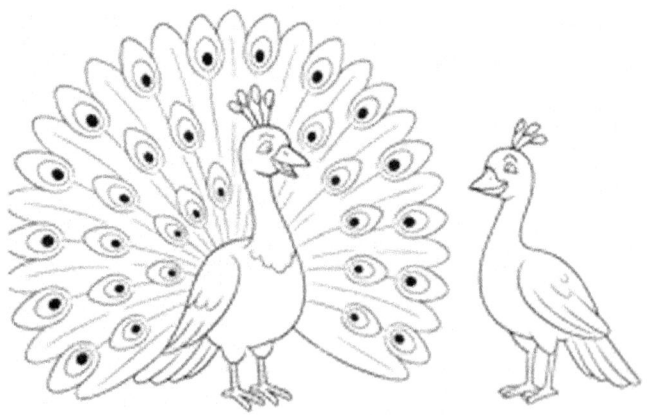

"À quoi penses-tu?"
(What are you thinking about?)

LET HER LOSE CONTROL BECAUSE YOU'RE FULLY IN YOURS

Dear Americans,

If you want her wild, you must be steady. Nothing makes a woman retreat faster than a man who laughs nervously, judges, or freezes when she lets herself go. But if you're grounded? She'll let the storm out. Her surrender isn't weakness—it's trust. And trust is the highest proof of desire. In France, we know: Her wildness is not chaos. It's her gift to you, the secret version of herself she only shows when she feels utterly safe. Hold your ground, and she'll shake the walls.

Comme on dit en France:
Elle est la tempête, mais toi tu dois être le phare.

As we say in France:
She is the storm, but you must be the lighthouse.

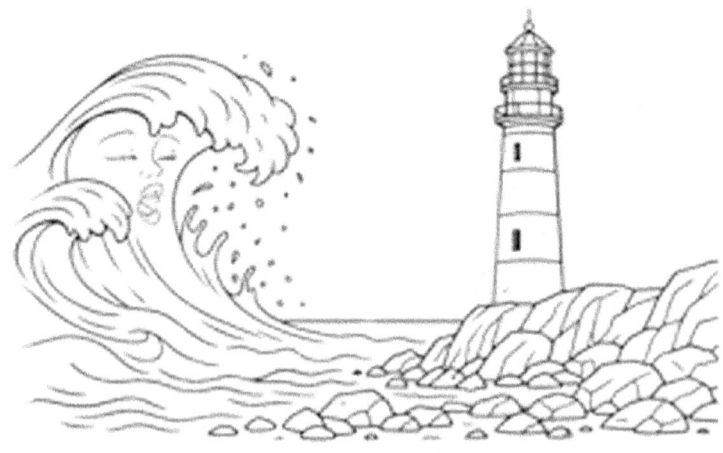

"À quoi penses-tu?"

(What are you thinking about?)

SHE DOESN'T WANT ROUTINE. SHE WANTS RITUAL

Dear Americans,

Rolling over like you're paying a utility bill is not seduction—it's laziness. Routine kills desire faster than fluorescent lighting. But ritual? Ritual is devotion. Dim the lights. Play music that wraps her in velvet. Set the sheets like a chef plating a dish. These aren't theatrics—they're signals: "You matter. This moment matters." In France, intimacy is treated like ceremony, not chores. Ritual doesn't overcomplicate passion—it elevates it. Routine is a clock. Ritual is a cathedral. Which do you think she'll remember?

Comme on dit en France:
Si tu veux l'electricite, appuie sur l'interrupteur.
Si tu veux la passion, allume des bougies.

As we say in France:
If you want electricity, flip a switch.
If you want passion, light candles.

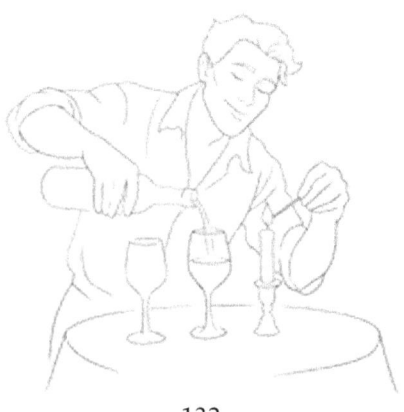

"À quoi penses-tu?"

(What are you thinking about?)

SMELL MATTERS MORE THAN SIZE

Dear Americans,

You can brag about stamina, angles, or size—but if your breath smells like garlic and your sheets like a locker room, it's over. Desire begins at the nose. Fresh skin, clean breath, maybe a whisper of cologne—that's what lingers. Neglect kills passion faster than bad technique. In France, we know that scent seduces before touch ever does. Sometimes the smallest detail—a trace of musk, soap, or skin—ignites fire more than inches ever could.

Comme on dit en France:
Parfois, c'est le nez qui guide plus que les yeux.

As we say in France:
Sometimes, it's the nose that leads more than the eyes.

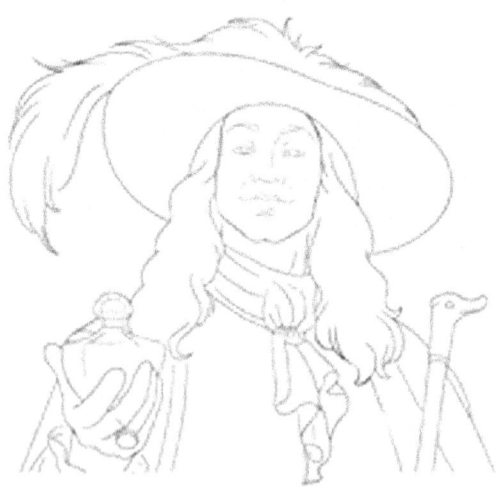

"À quoi penses-tu?"

(What are you thinking about?)

DON'T JUST TOUCH HER.
LET HER TOUCH YOU, TOO

Dear Americans,

Stop acting like sex is a one-man performance. Let her join the orchestra. Let her grip your back, pull your hips, map your chest. Let her see your breath stutter; let her hear you moan. In France, intimacy is a duet, not a monologue. Yes, giving is sexy. But allowing her to take? That's when passion becomes poetry. Be her canvas, let her paint with fire. When two lovers create together, desire doesn't double—it multiplies.

Comme on dit en France:
L'amour n'est pas un solo, c'est un duo.

As we say in France:
Love is not a solo—it's a duet.

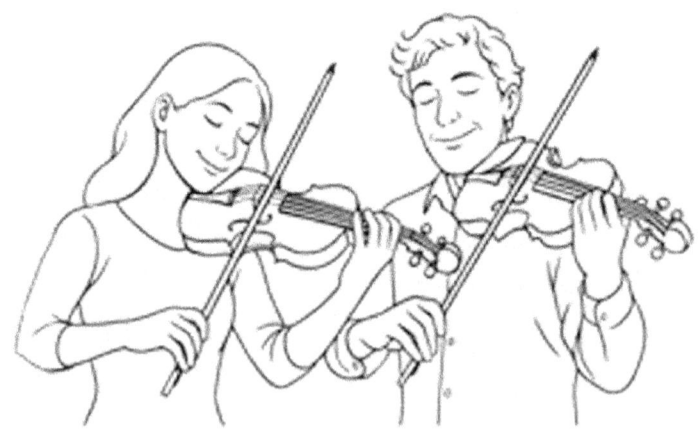

"À quoi penses-tu?"

(What are you thinking about?)

TEASE HER MIND
BEFORE YOU UNDRESS HER BODY

Dear Americans,

If you wait until the bedroom, you're already late. Seduction starts in the morning—an outrageous whisper over coffee, a bold text at noon, a stolen glance in the evening. By nightfall, she's been simmering for hours. That's foreplay—the kind that doesn't need a timer. In France, we know anticipation is the spice of passion. A single word, well-placed, can make her body crave you before your hands arrive.

Comme on dit en France:
Le désir commence souvent par un mot bien placé.

As we say in France:
Desire often begins with a well-placed word.

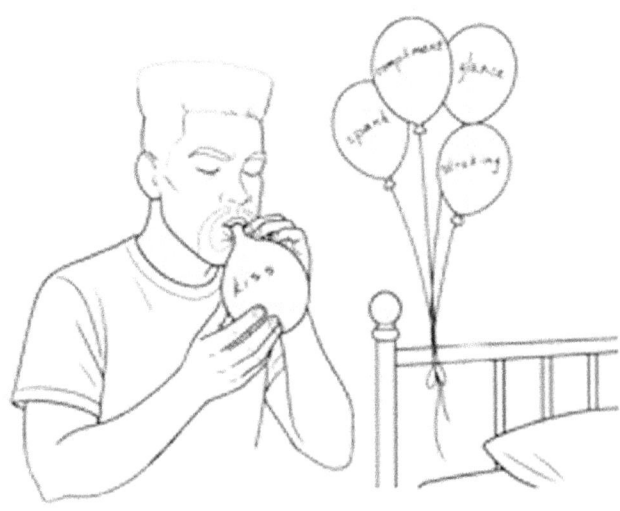

"À quoi penses-tu?"

(What are you thinking about?)

HER BODY IS NOT
AN OBSTACLE COURSE

Dear Americans,

Stop treating her like she's a video game with levels to unlock. She's not an obstacle course—she's a universe. Every curve, every sigh is not a checkpoint but an invitation. Don't sprint. Wander. Explore like a Frenchman strolling through Paris: unhurried, curious, intoxicated by detail. The orgasm is not a trophy; the journey is the art. In France, we don't race to the finish line; we savor the landscape of pleasure, step by step, as if it never ends.

Comme on dit en France:
L'amour n'est pas un sprint, mais une promenade éternelle.

As we say in France:
Love is not a sprint, but an endless stroll.

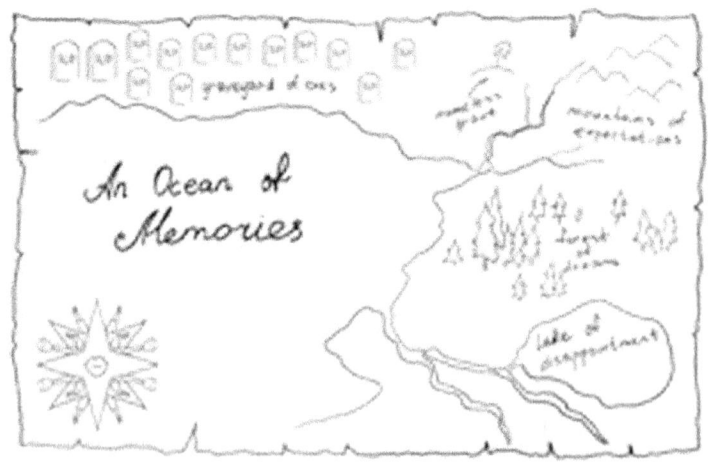

"À quoi penses-tu?"
(What are you thinking about?)

DON'T BE AFRAID TO BE TENDER

Dear Americans,

You think tenderness is weakness? Non. It's the ultimate proof of strength. Hold her when she cries, laugh with her when life cracks her open, stay when the storm comes. Muscles impress at the gym; tenderness seduces in the bedroom. A woman doesn't remember your bench press—she remembers the arms that wrapped her when the world fell apart. In France, we know: The harder the world outside, the softer she longs for you inside. That's not weakness, that's mastery.

Comme on dit en France:
La tendresse est la plus grande preuve de force.

As we say in France:
Tenderness is the greatest proof of strength.

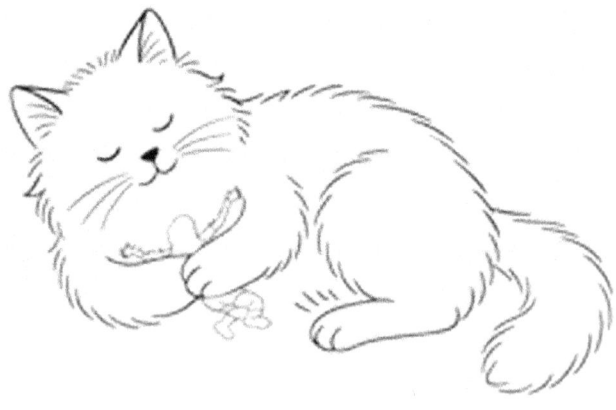

"À quoi penses-tu?"
(What are you thinking about?)

THE BEST LOVERS ARE CURIOUS, NOT COCKY

Dear Americans,

Confidence is sexy, arrogance is boring. Stop arriving like you've got a PhD in women. You don't. Every woman is a new country with a different language. Some require translation, others improvisation. The greatest lovers aren't cocky—they're curious. They ask, they listen, they explore. "Show me..." is infinitely hotter than "I know." In France, we know the most seductive lovers act like travelers, not tour guides. Curiosity isn't weakness; it's elegance.

Comme on dit en France:
La curiosité est l'élégance du désir.

As we say in France:
Curiosity is the elegance of desire.

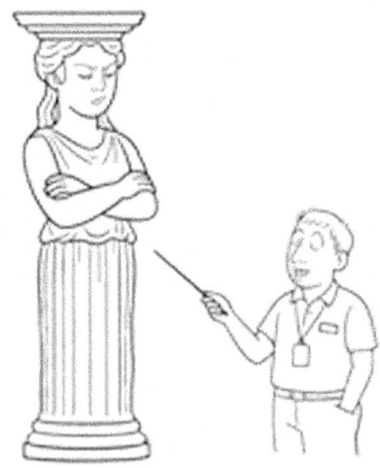

"À quoi penses-tu?"

(What are you thinking about?)

THERE'S NO "RIGHT WAY" TO MAKE LOVE

Dear Americans,

You love manuals, IKEA desks, iPhones, even sex. But guess what? There's no universal instruction sheet for making love. What thrills one-woman bores another. What works tonight might fail tomorrow. Great lovers don't chase formulas—they chase connection. Desire is jazz, not classical, improvisation, not rigid notes. In France, we know passion is alive, unpredictable, deliciously unstable. Forget the recipe. Pay attention. Be curious. The only "right way" is the way that makes her eyes close, and her breath catch.

Comme on dit en France:
La passion n'a pas de mode d'emploi.

As we say in France:
Passion doesn't come with a manual.

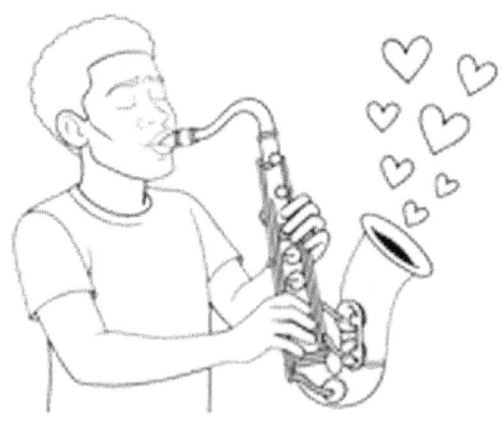

"À quoi penses-tu?"

(What are you thinking about?)

GREAT LOVERS ASK, THEY DON'T ASSUME

Dear Americans,

Assumption is the enemy of intimacy. Too many men climb into bed like know-it-alls. Wrong. The most seductive move isn't your hand; it's your voice. Not porn talk, but curiosity: "Do you like this?" "Do you want more?" These questions aren't weak. They're electric. They say, "I want to know you." In France, we don't pretend we have the answers—we ask better questions. Because desire doesn't begin in the hips, it begins in the ears.

Comme on dit en France:
Le désir commence par une question, pas une position.

As we say in France:
Desire begins with a question, not a position.

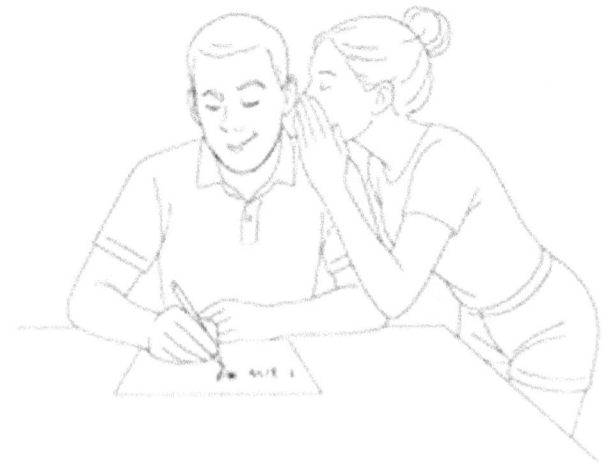

"À quoi penses-tu?"

(What are you thinking about?)

EXPLORATION IS THE NEW SEDUCTION

Dear Americans,

Stop trying to be experts. Be explorers. Every woman is uncharted territory. Every sigh is a map, every tremor a compass. Touch like a traveler, not a conqueror. Let her body teach you; let curiosity guide you. In France, we know the real thrill isn't mastery, it's mystery. You don't become a lover by memorizing techniques—you become one by discovering her. Slowly. Patiently. Like savoring a new wine.

Comme on dit en France:
C'est en explorant qu'on devient amant.

As we say in France:
It is by exploring that one becomes a lover.

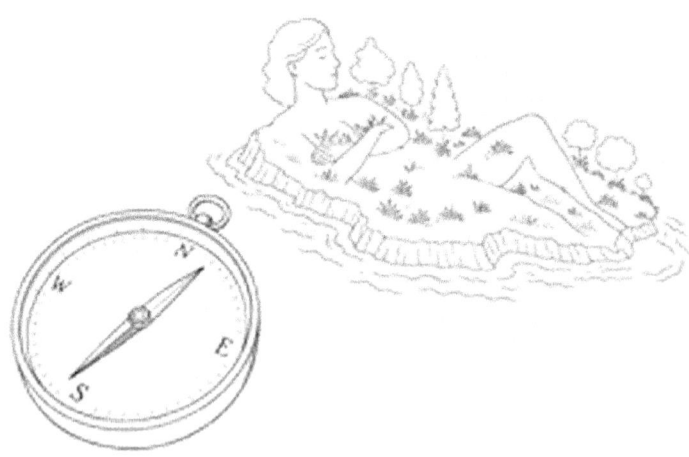

"À quoi penses-tu?"

(What are you thinking about?)

WITHOUT SAFETY, THERE IS NO SURRENDER

Dear Americans,

If she stiffens when you touch her, the problem isn't her—it's you. Or more precisely, the space you've created. Desire doesn't bloom in tension; it blooms in trust. No candle or lingerie will matter if she doesn't feel safe. But when she does? Mon Dieu. She lets go. Entirely. Passion without safety is fragile. Passion with safety? Explosive. In France, we know the most powerful aphrodisiac isn't lace or wine—it's reassurance.

Comme on dit en France:
Un cœur en sécurité ouvre un corps sans effort.

As we say in France:
A safe heart opens a body without effort.

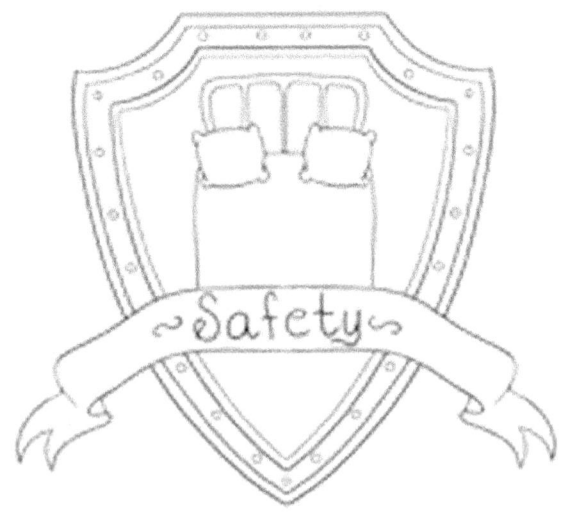

"À quoi penses-tu?"
(What are you thinking about?)

AGE ISN'T AN EXPIRATION DATE

Dear Americans,

You treat passion like it comes with a warranty—valid until forty, maybe fifty, then poof. Non! Desire doesn't retire. The skin may wrinkle, but the heart still sprints when touched. The body changes, yes, but the fire inside? It refuses to check a calendar. In France, we don't ask, "Am I too old for love?" We ask, "Why would I stop now?" Age doesn't shrink passion—it makes it more delicious, more intentional, freer.

Comme on dit en France:
Le cœur ne vieillit pas, il bat juste plus sage.

As we say in France:
The heart doesn't age—it simply beats wiser.

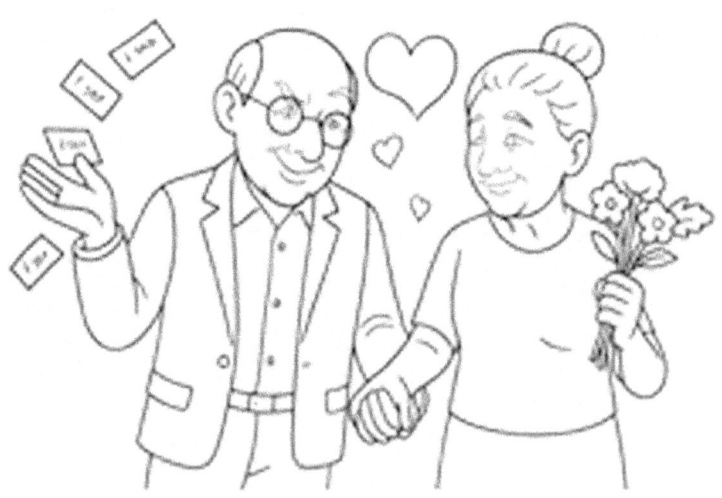

"À quoi penses-tu?"

(What are you thinking about?)

THE LIBIDO DOESN'T COLLECT SOCIAL SECURITY

Dear Americans,

Retirement checks may come, but passion doesn't stand in line at the post office. Some of the best sex happens after sixty. Why? Less stress, fewer insecurities, more presence. At thirty, you rush. At seventy, you savor. The world slows, but intimacy deepens. French lovers know real pleasure comes when you finally stop pretending, you're in a competition. Retirement doesn't mean abstinence—it means liberation.

Comme on dit en France:
Moins de stress, plus de caresses.

As we say in France:
Less stress, more caress.

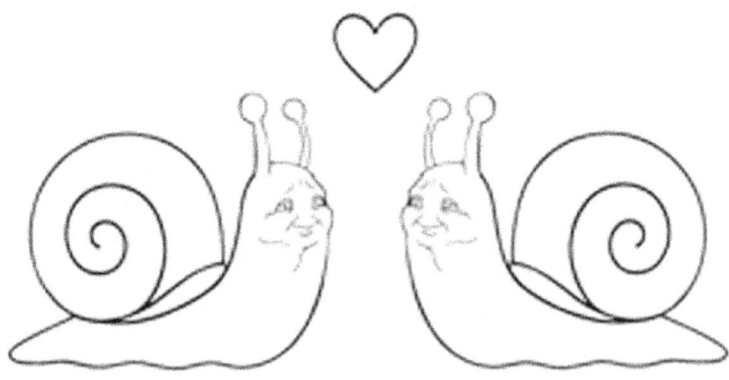

"À quoi penses-tu?"

(What are you thinking about?)

GRAY HAIR, GOLDEN NIGHTS

Dear Americans,

You see gray hair as decline. In France, we see it as a crown. Silver on the head often means gold between the sheets. With age comes confidence, clarity, and the courage to say exactly what you want without blushing. No games, no guessing— just honesty wrapped in experience. The young have stamina, maybe. The mature have mastery. And believe me, mastery wins.

Comme on dit en France:
Argent sur la tête, or entre les draps.

As we say in France:
Silver on the head, gold between the sheets.

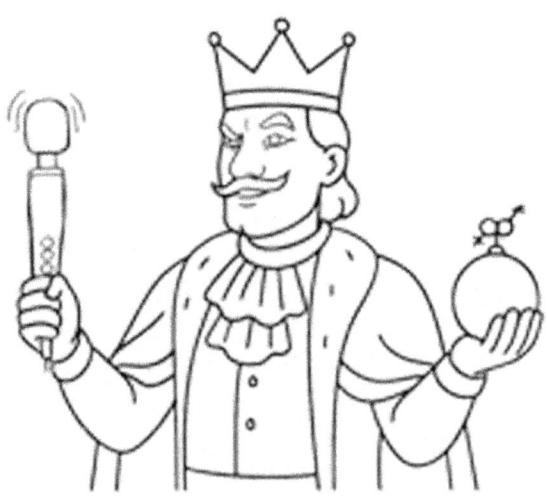

"À quoi penses-tu?"

(What are you thinking about?)

THE BEDROOM IS NOT JUST FOR THE YOUNG

Dear Americans,

Who sold you the lie that sex is for gymnasts under thirty? Intimacy doesn't require acrobatics—it requires connection. At twenty, you move fast. At sixty, you move right. Tenderness, patience, attention—these grow with age, and they make passion deeper than any youthful tumble. Love isn't a sport; it's an art. And art gets better with time.

Comme on dit en France:
Ce n'est pas l'âge, c'est l'appétit.

As we say in France:
It's not the age—it's the appetite.

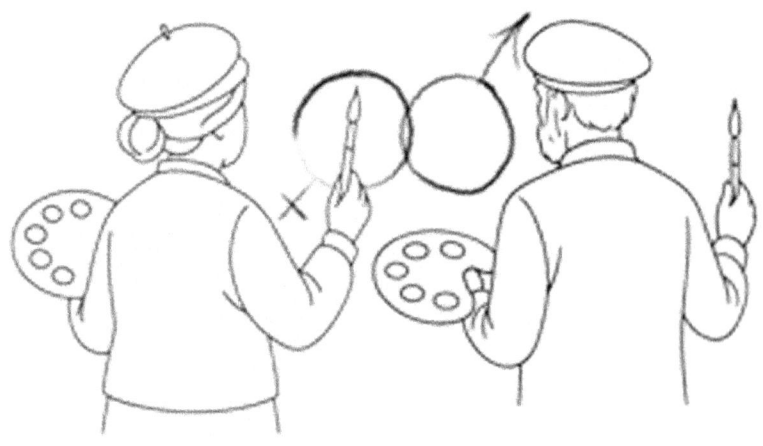

"À quoi penses-tu?"

(What are you thinking about?)

PRESCRIPTION FOR PLEASURE

Dear Americans,

Yes, sometimes there are blood pressure meds, arthritis creams, or the famous little blue pill. But don't confuse adjustments with absence. Desire is alive—it just comes with better playlists, extra pillows, and maybe bifocals. And honestly? That only makes it funnier, warmer, freer. French lovers know a little help doesn't kill the fire—it fuels it.

Comme on dit en France:
Un petit coup de pouce n'a jamais arrêté une grande performance.

As we say in France:
A little help never stopped a great performance.

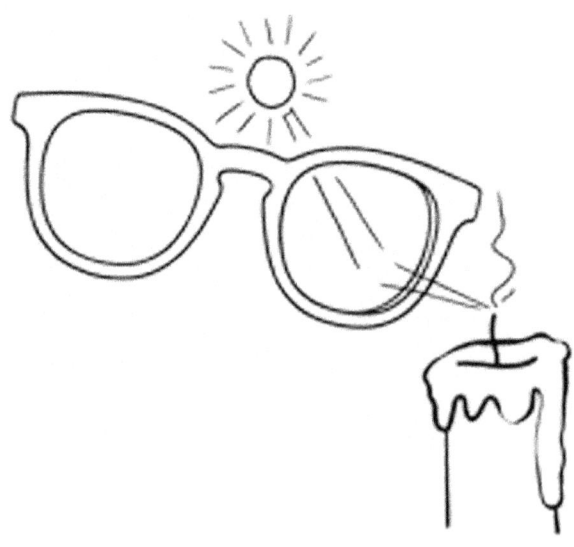

162

"À quoi penses-tu?"

(What are you thinking about?)

THEY'RE STILL DOING IT (THEY'RE JUST NOT POSTING ABOUT IT)

Dear Americans,

Older couples don't flaunt passion online and thank God for that. No selfies. No hashtags. Just quiet, unfiltered intimacy behind closed doors. Some of the hottest love stories happen where nobody is watching. Real fire doesn't need a stage—it just needs two willing bodies and a little privacy. France understands this well: Intimacy isn't performance, it's presence.

Comme on dit en France:
Le vrai feu n'a pas besoin de public.

As we say in France:
True fire doesn't need an audience.

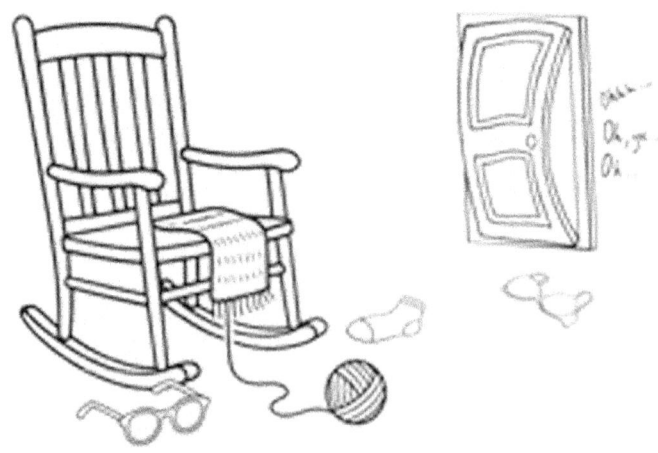

"À quoi penses-tu?"

(What are you thinking about?)

SENSUALITY GETS BETTER WITH AGE

Dear Americans,

You think passion belongs to the young? Non. Older lovers know the secret: Slow is sexy. They understand foreplay isn't the appetizer—it's the whole feast. Eye contact lingers, kisses deepen, touches turn into poetry. With age, speed loses value, but savoring becomes irresistible. What was once a race becomes a dance. The climax is no longer the prize—the connection is. And connection, my friends, never wrinkles.

Comme on dit en France:
Lent, c'est le nouveau sexy.

As we say in France:
Slow is the new sexy.

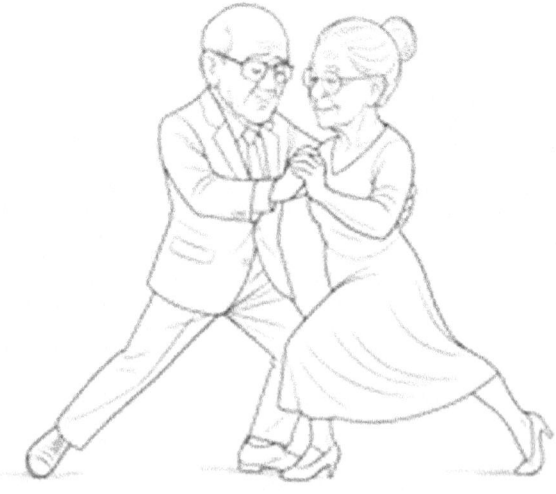

"À quoi penses-tu?"

(What are you thinking about?)

RETIREMENT DOESN'T MEAN RESIGNATION

Dear Americans,

When the kids leave and the house goes quiet, many couples rediscover the bed like it's Paris in spring. Retirement isn't resignation—it's revelation. With fewer deadlines and more free mornings, passion sneaks back in, carrying coffee and mischief. Lovers see each other again, not as chauffeurs or coworkers, but as partners, explorers, conspirators. Freedom brings fire, and silence makes room for whispers. Believe me, many sixty-year-olds are busier under the sheets than twenty-year-olds on dating apps.

Comme on dit en France:
L'amour revient quand le bruit s'en va.

As we say in France:
Love often returns when the noise leaves.

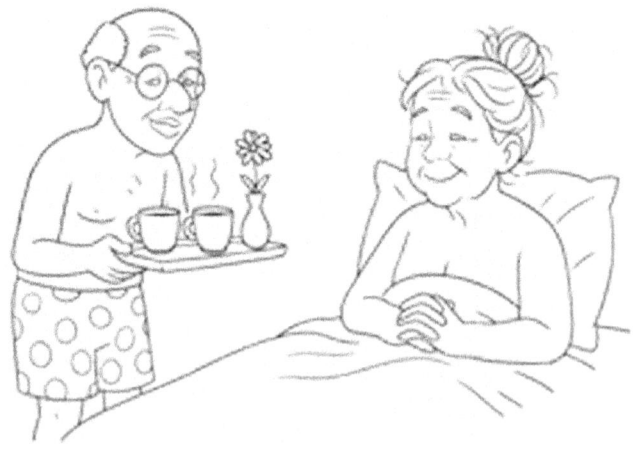

"À quoi penses-tu?"

(What are you thinking about?)

DESIRE DOESN'T CHECK BIRTHDAYS

Dear Americans,

Desire doesn't retire with your candles. Lust doesn't pack up after fifty. If anything, it grows sharper, funnier, freer. Wrinkles don't kill attraction—they give it character. The hunger for touch, for laughter, for fire, never dies. The only thing that changes is how you savor it. Youth bring speed; age brings spice. The French know passion has no passport, no schedule, no shame. It ages like wine—the older, the deeper, the better.

Comme on dit en France:
La passion n'a ni passeport, ni date de péremption.

As we say in France:
Passion has no passport, no expiration date.

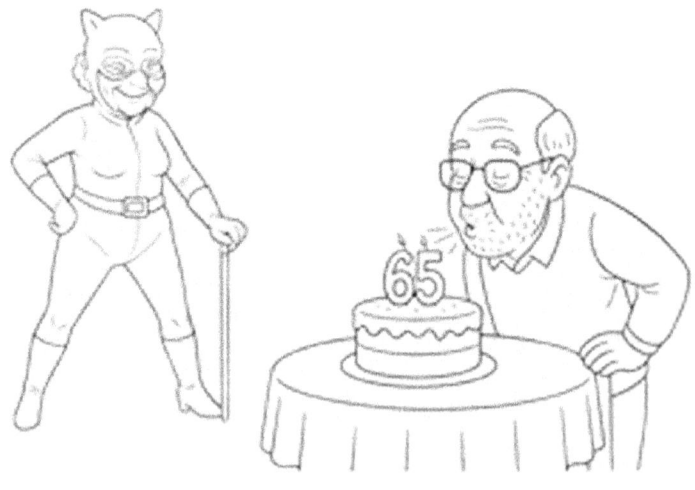

"À quoi penses-tu?"

(What are you thinking about?)

THINKS FILTHY LANGUAGE IS A PERSONALITY

Dear Americans,

Dropping "f***" every two words isn't edgy—it's lazy. Vulgarity isn't depth; it's camouflage for insecurity. Anyone can bark filth, but it takes real charm to seduce with wit, timing, and restraint. Crude noise fades, but a clever phrase lingers in the heart. French lovers know the sharpest dagger and the softest caress are both hidden in words. When chosen well, they melt her faster than any profanity ever could.

Comme on dit en France:
Les mots crus n'ont jamais fait fondre un cœur.

As we say in France:
Crude words have never melted a heart.

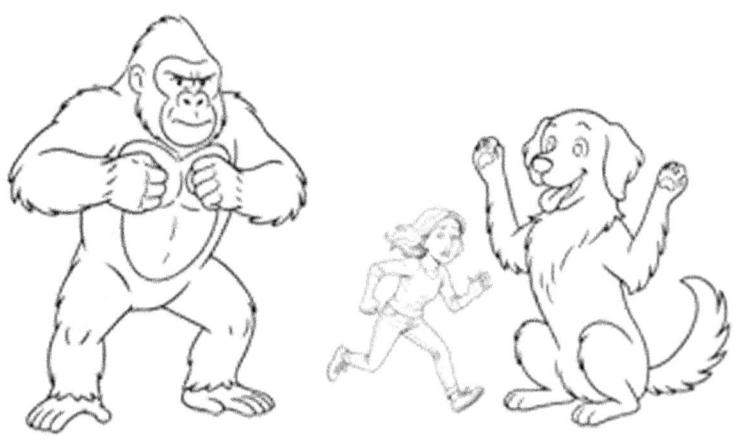

"À quoi penses-tu?"

(What are you thinking about?)

MANSPREADING TO ASSERT DOMINANCE

Dear Americans,

Let's be clear: spreading your knees two ZIP codes apart doesn't make you powerful—it makes you ridiculous. You're not a king on a throne; you're a man on public transport. Confidence isn't measured in inches of subway real estate; it's measured in presence, in calm, in how safe others feel around you. Real power is graceful, not greedy. The French know: Seduction is not domination—it's consideration.

Comme on dit en France:
Le vrai pouvoir, c'est laisser de la place à l'autre.

As we say in France:
True power is making space for the other.

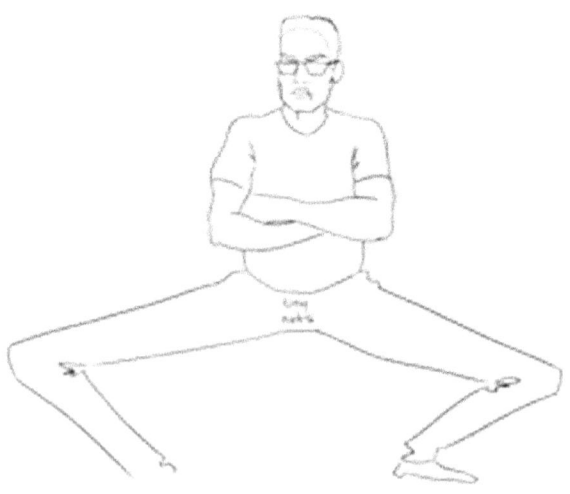

"À quoi penses-tu?"
(What are you thinking about?)

THE "ALPHA" CRUTCH

Dear Americans,

If you must shout, "I'm alpha," trust me, you're not. Real leaders don't wear hashtags; they wear calm. Masculinity isn't volume—it's gravity. The louder the roar, the more fragile the ego. In France, we laugh at the "alpha" label because confidence doesn't need an introduction. Presence speaks louder than posturing, and groundedness seduces more than growling ever will.

Comme on dit en France:
Plus tu cries fort, moins tu impressionnes.

As we say in France:
The louder you yell, the less you impress.

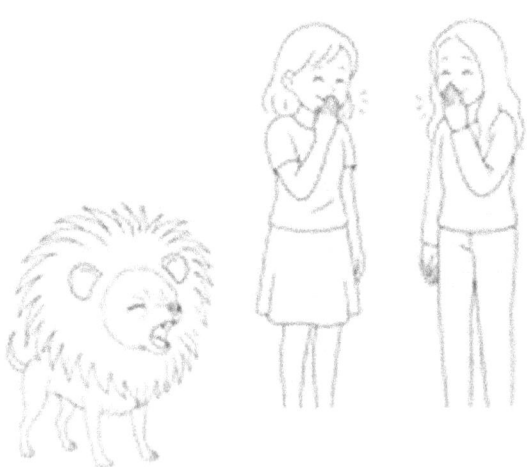

"À quoi penses-tu?"
(What are you thinking about?)

MAIN CHARACTER SYNDROME

Dear Americans,

If you treat waiters, strangers, or even your wife like extras in your movie, you've already lost the plot. Charm is not something you perform on date night—it's how you treat everyone, every day. In France, seduction is a lifestyle, not an act. Politeness at the café, courtesy on the street, tenderness at home—this is the charisma that lingers. Everyday decency, not cinematic drama, is what makes a man unforgettable.

Comme on dit en France:
Le charme commence avec la courtoisie.

As we say in France:
Charm begins with courtesy.

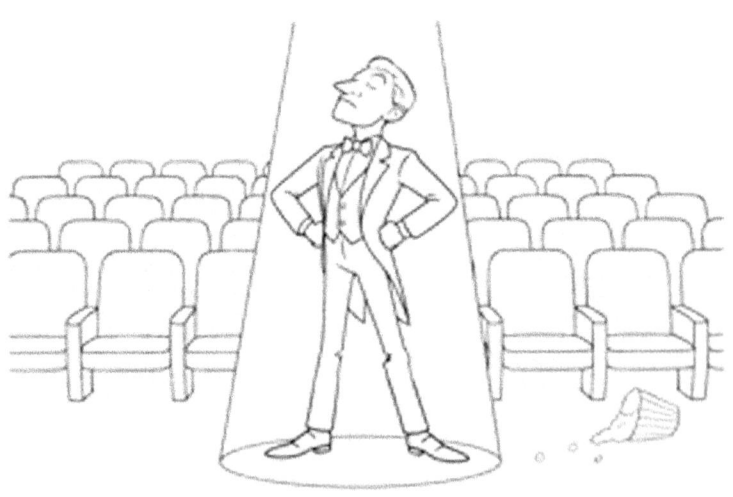

"À quoi penses-tu?"

(What are you thinking about?)

THERAPY?
HE THINKS IT'S A JOKE

Dear Americans,

"Just chill," he says while she's in tears. But the truth? He's terrified of facing himself. Therapy isn't weakness—it's literacy in the language of emotions. Mocking therapy is like mocking reading when you can't spell. In France, we know courage is looking inward, not running away. You can't heal what you won't name. Emotional cowardice, not therapy, is the epidemic.

Comme on dit en France:
Tu ne peux pas guérir ce que tu refuses de nommer.

As we say in France:
You can't heal what you refuse to name.

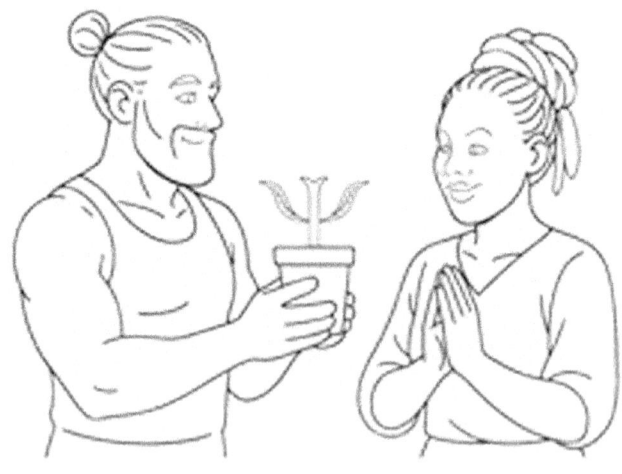

"À quoi penses-tu?"

(What are you thinking about?)

ALLERGIC TO 'PLEASE' AND 'THANK YOU'? NON, MERCI.

Dear Americans,

If he can't thank the waitress, don't expect him to thank his wife. Gratitude isn't optional—it's oxygen. Politeness doesn't make you soft; it makes you magnetic. Arrogance kills desire faster than bad breath. French lovers know simple manners— "s'il vous plaît, merci"—are the sexiest soundtrack to daily life. Politeness never goes out of style, but entitlement never comes into fashion.

Comme on dit en France:
Un homme poli n'est jamais démodé.

As we say in France:
A well-mannered man is never out of style.

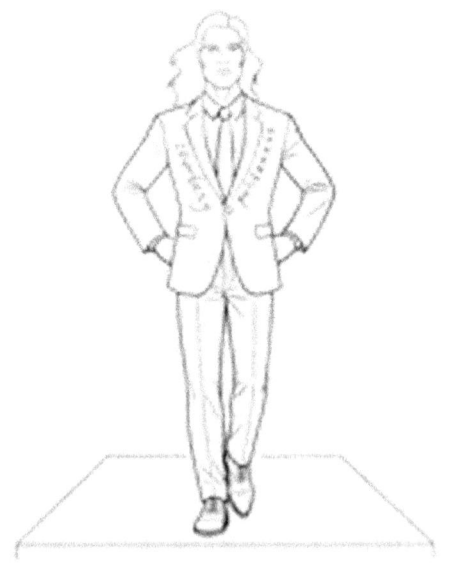

"À quoi penses-tu?"

(What are you thinking about?)

INTIMACY DIES
WHERE RESPECT DISAPPEARS

Dear Americans,

Sex doesn't vanish first. Appreciation does. When gratitude is gone, when respect is replaced by sarcasm or silence, intimacy is the next casualty. You can't expect kisses when the day is full of cold shoulders. In France, we never forget compliments are not optional—they are oxygen. A woman who feels unseen won't open. A man who feels disrespected won't chase. Desire doesn't collapse overnight—it starves slowly from neglect.

Comme on dit en France:
"L'absence de respect tue l'envie avant l'absence de désir."

As we say in France:
Disrespect kills desire before desire ever dies.

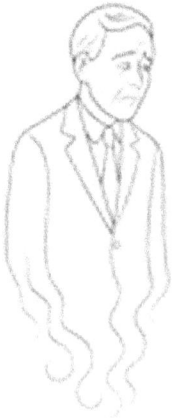
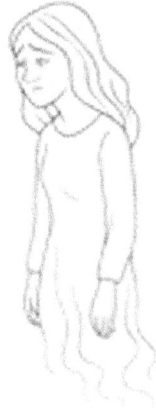

"À quoi penses-tu?"
(What are you thinking about?)

INTIMACY IS THE BAROMETER, NOT THE ENGINE

Dear Americans,

You think sex will fix everything—Non. Sex is not the engine of love; it's the barometer. It reflects the climate of your marriage. If respect fades, if gratitude disappears, the forecast is cold sheets and closed bodies. Desire doesn't collapse overnight; it starves when appreciation vanishes, and sarcasm takes its place. In France, we know compliments are not decoration—they are fuel. A partner who feels seen opens like a flower; one who feels dismissed withers. The bedroom only thrives when kindness precedes it.

And if you think sex alone will fix disrespect—mon ami, that's like trying to patch a sinking boat with a condom.

Comme on dit en France:
Le respect nourrit le désir.

As we say in France:
Respect feeds desire.

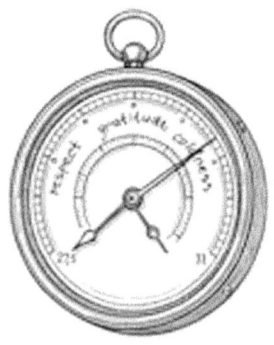

"À quoi penses-tu?"

(What are you thinking about?)

LACK OF APPRECIATION KILLS DESIRE BEFORE THE BEDROOM

Dear Americans,

You think intimacy fades because of age or stress. Non. Intimacy fades because disrespect moves in first. Lack of appreciation is the silent assassin of desire. Criticism, sarcasm, or simply ignoring each other—these daily poisons kill passion long before the lights go out. You can't expect fireworks in bed when you are cold outside of it. In France, we know gratitude is not optional—it's lubrication for love. A "thank you" can ignite more fire than lingerie. Desire doesn't begin in the sheets—it begins with respect at the dinner table.

Comme on dit en France:
Le mépris éteint plus de lits que la fatigue.

As we say in France:
Contempt kills more bedrooms than fatigue.

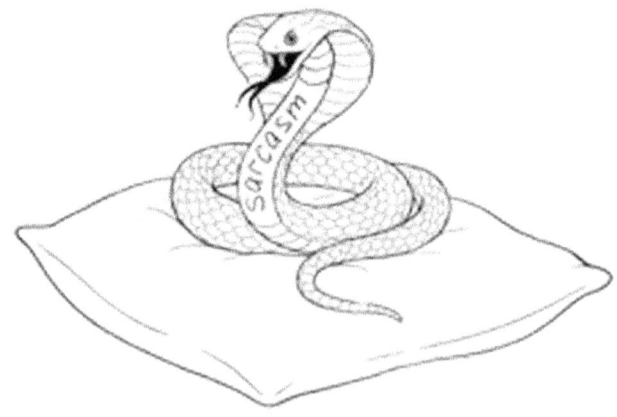

"À quoi penses-tu?"
(What are you thinking about?)

A SEXLESS MARRIAGE IS JUST A CONTRACT, NOT A CONNECTION

Dear Americans,

A sexless marriage is not really a marriage—it's an arrangement. A quiet pact to coexist without touching. You eat together, sleep beside each other, raise kids... but the fire is gone. One partner says, "I tried talking." The other says nothing. And silence becomes the agreement. In France, we know desire is not optional—it is the lifeblood of love. Without it, you're not lovers, just roommates with paperwork. If the bed stays cold, the heart eventually walks. Intimacy isn't extra—it's the proof of marriage itself.

Comme on dit en France:
Un mariage sans désir est un contrat sans âme.

As we say in France:
A marriage without desire is a contract without a soul.

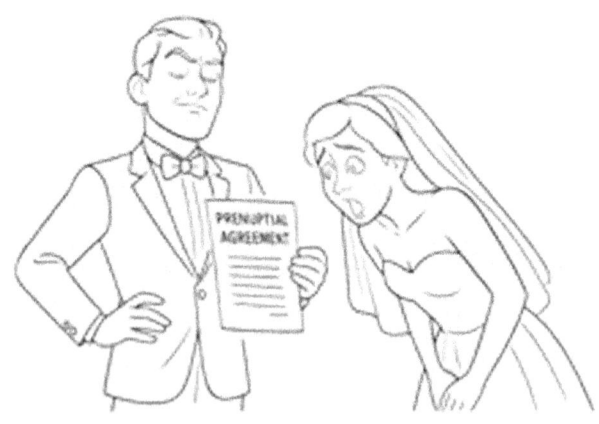

"À quoi penses-tu?"

(What are you thinking about?)

A SEXLESS MARRIAGE
IS DIVORCE IN DISGUISE

Dear Americans,

A sexless marriage is not peace—it's purgatory. You tell yourselves you're "fine," but the silence in the bedroom is louder than any argument. No kisses, no touches, no fire… just routine dressed up as commitment. In France, we'd call it what it is: a divorce not yet finalized. Because without intimacy, you're not lovers—you're administrators of a shared mortgage. Passion is not a luxury; it's the proof you're still married. Kill the fire, and you're just negotiating terms until one of you finally leaves.

Comme on dit en France:
Sans désir, le mariage est déjà mort.

As we say in France:
Without desire, the marriage is already dead.

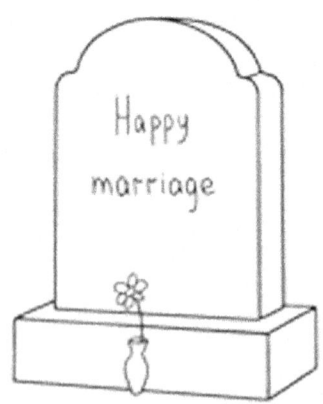

"À quoi penses-tu?"

(What are you thinking about?)

ATTENTION ISN'T AFFECTION

Dear Americans,

It amazes me how many American women confuse sexual attention with being truly wanted. A man may undress you with his eyes, but that doesn't mean he wants your heart. Lust can be cheap—it costs him nothing. Commitment, admiration, devotion? That's the rare currency. In France, we know the difference: Sex without affection is just appetite. Real desire isn't only about having your body—it's about wanting your presence, your laugh, your chaos, your calm. Don't mistake the spotlight of attention for the warmth of love. One burns out. The other stays lit.

Comme on dit en France:
Le désir n'est pas toujours l'amour.

As we say in France:
Desire is not always love.

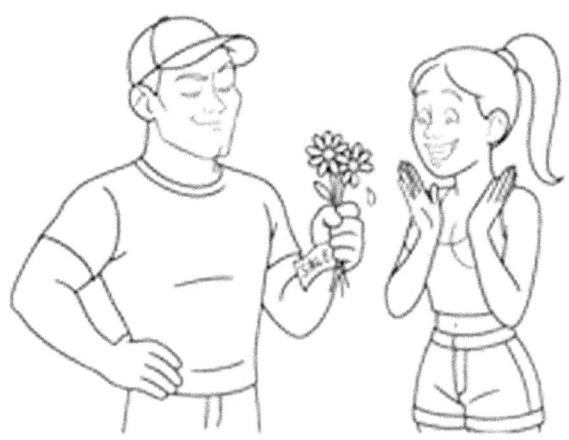

"À quoi penses-tu?"
(What are you thinking about?)

ATTRACTION IS THE GATEKEEPER

Dear Americans,

No love story ever began without attraction. Chemistry isn't optional—it's the entry ticket. Desire comes first, and then the woman decides if the spark becomes fire. Men may chase, but women choose. That's not weakness—it's sovereignty. In France, we don't deny this law of nature. You can't argue your way into lust. You either spark it—or you don't. Everything else—love, marriage, forever—is built on that first undeniable flame.

And if you think swiping right without spark will save you—bonne chance, you're not dating, you're just shopping.

Comme on dit en France:
Pas d'attirance, pas de danse.

As we say in France:
No attraction, no dance.

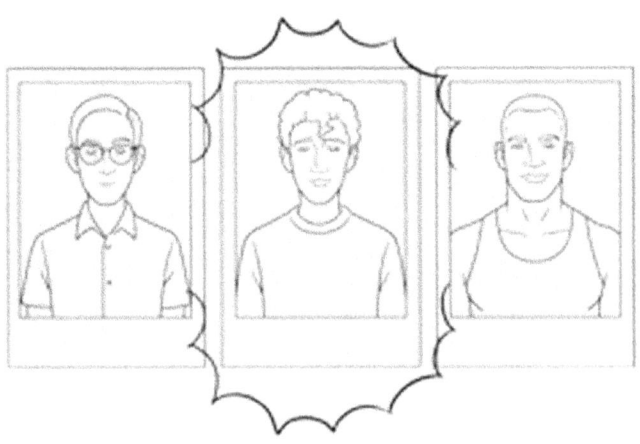

"À quoi penses-tu?"
(What are you thinking about?)

DESIRE IS NOT ONE-SIDED

Dear Americans,

How some women think they can lose interest and then declare the bedroom closed—while expecting the man to stay celibate—is beyond me. Marriage is not a monastery. Desire is a two-way street, not a ration card. If you lock the doors of intimacy, don't be shocked when love escapes through the window. In France, we don't treat passion like an optional subscription you can cancel at will. If the fire fades, you rebuild it together—you don't punish each other with starvation.

Comme on dit en France:
Le lit n'est pas une prison, c'est un jardin.

As we say in France:
The bed is not a prison—it's a garden.

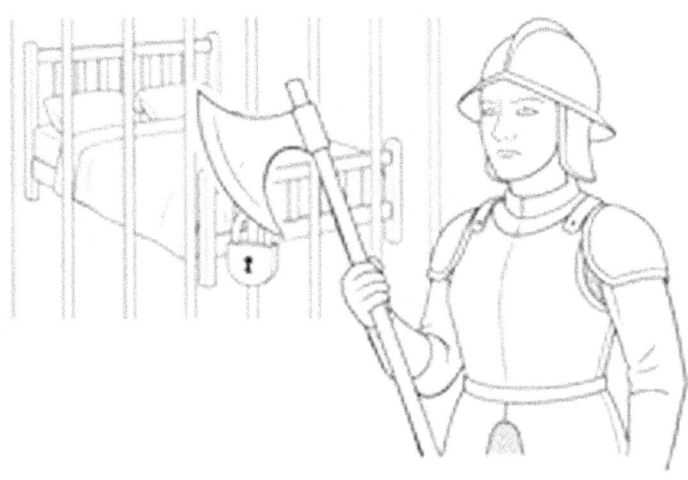

"À quoi penses-tu?"

(What are you thinking about?)

TRUTH #100

MY WAY OR NO WAY KILLS THE HIGHWAY

Dear Americans,

Some women mistake marriage for a dictatorship: my way or the highway. But a bed is not a battlefield, and intimacy is not a hostage situation. Twenty years without touch? That isn't partnership—it's punishment. Love cannot survive on ultimatums. Desire needs freedom, play, and give-and-take. In France, we know: The moment intimacy becomes a weapon, it stops being love. A man is not a monk, and a wife is not a warden. The bedroom should unite, not imprison.

Comme on dit en France:
Quand l'amour devient une arme, il cesse d'être de l'amour.

As we say in France:
When love becomes a weapon, it ceases to be love.

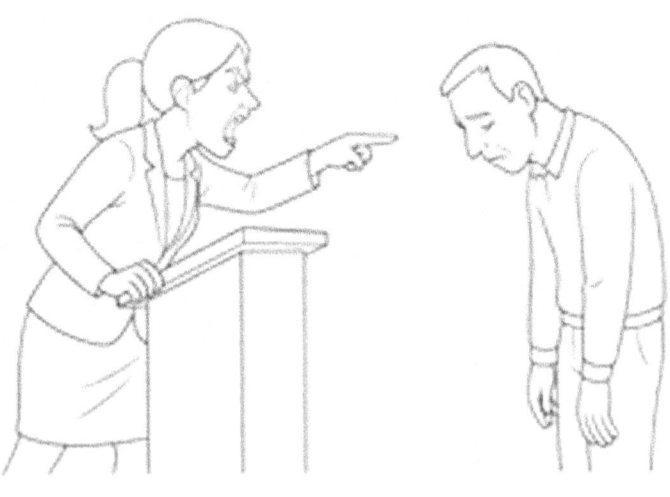

"À quoi penses-tu?"
(What are you thinking about?)

DESIRE DOESN'T RETIRE AT 50

Dear Americans,

Older men get shamed for dating younger women, but let's be honest: Men don't lose their sex drive at fifty. Many still burn like they did at thirty. The problem? Too many women his age have turned intimacy into a museum piece—look but don't touch. So why is he the villain for seeking passion where it still lives? Younger women often adore older men precisely for their confidence, presence, and experience. In France, we don't blame the hungry man—we ask why the kitchen went cold.

Comme on dit en France:
On ne blâme pas celui qui a faim, mais celui qui ferme la cuisine.

As we say in France:
Don't blame the hungry man—blame the one who closed the kitchen.

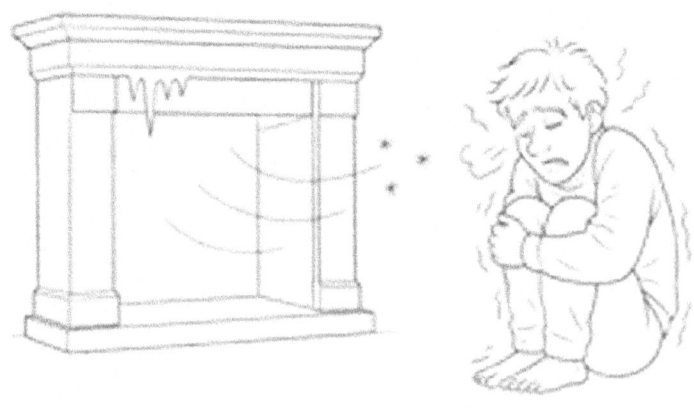

"À quoi penses-tu?"

(What are you thinking about?)

TRUTH #102

WHEN SEX DIES, SOMETHING DEEPER IS ALREADY SICK

Dear Americans,

Sexless marriages are rarely about schedules or hormones—it's often about pathology. When one partner shuts down emotionally, humor vanishes, effort fades, and intimacy becomes rationed like bread in wartime. The bedroom is only the final symptom. A healthy lover leans in, but a damaged one withdraws, treating sex as an obligation or manipulation. In France, we know laughter, touch, and passion all come from the same flame. When intimacy ends, it's not just desire that's gone—it's health. Don't ignore it. Absence in bed is often the autopsy of a dying relationship.

Comme on dit en France:
Quand le lit se tait, le cœur est déjà malade.

As we say in France:
When the bed goes silent, the heart is already sick.

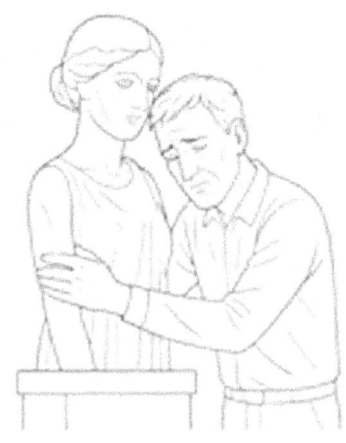

"À quoi penses-tu?"

(What are you thinking about?)

THE CRUELEST AFFAIR IS ONE WITH INDIFFERENCE

Dear Americans,

Sex inside marriage should be the most beautiful proof of love—but when one partner stops "seeing" the other, it becomes the cruelest heartbreak. A wife can endure wrinkles, bills, even storms—but not invisibility. Nothing crushes the soul more than lying beside someone whose eyes are always elsewhere. Desire doesn't die from age; it dies from neglect. In France, we say passion isn't about looking around—it's about looking deeper at the same person, every day. True intimacy is not variety—it's devotion.

Comme on dit en France:
L'infidélité commence quand les yeux s'éloignent du cœur.

As we say in France:
Infidelity begins when the eyes drift from the heart.

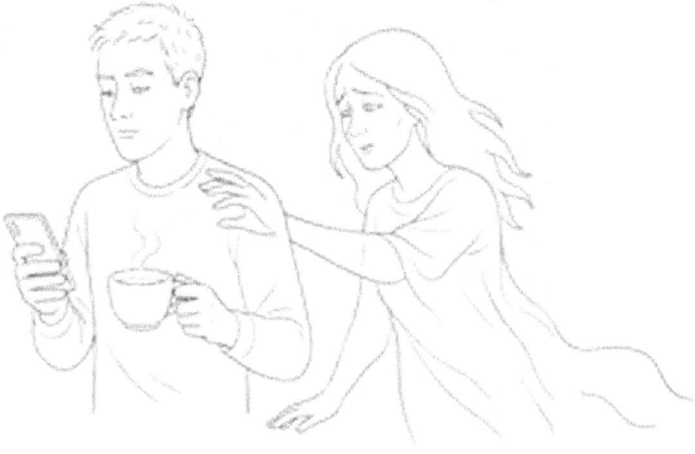

"À quoi penses-tu?"

(What are you thinking about?)

MENOPAUSE ISN'T A PAUSE BUTTON

Dear Americans,

Some men joke that "menopause" means they've been put on pause. Non. It's not a stop sign—it's a shift. The music doesn't end; it just changes tempo. If you act like desire is dead, you'll become the bored man on the couch waiting for "regular programming" to return. In France, we see menopause as a new act, not the curtain call. Treat her like a mystery still unfolding, not a machine that's out of warranty. That's how you discover fire that burns deeper, not weaker.

Comme on dit en France:
Ce n'est pas une panne, c'est une métamorphose.

As we say in France:
It's not a breakdown—it's a metamorphosis.

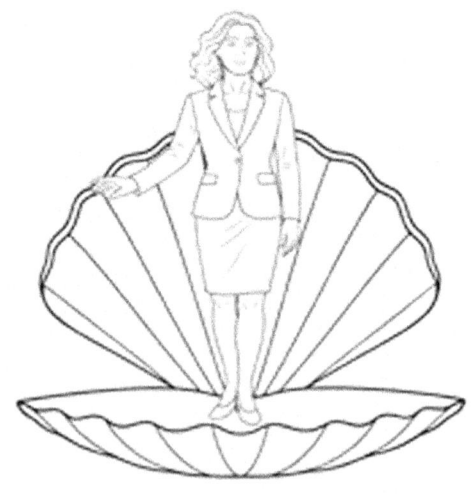

"À quoi penses-tu?"

(What are you thinking about?)

TRUTH #105

LOSING SEX
MEANS LOSING THE MARRIAGE

Dear Americans,

Some marriages don't end with papers—they end when the bed goes cold. I've seen couples choose food, TV, and silence over passion, and then wonder why everything else collapsed. Sex isn't just recreation—it's connection, renewal, proof you're still choosing each other. When intimacy dies, resentment grows fat even faster than the waistline. Better to walk away with nothing than stay with someone who offers you everything but themselves. Desire doesn't retire with age—it retires when neglected. And those who keep it alive know life is much sweeter.

Comme on dit en France:
Quand le lit meurt, le mariage suit.

As we say in France:
When the bed dies, the marriage follows.

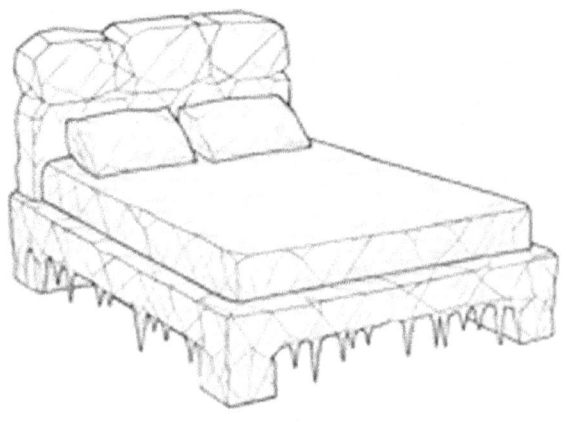

"À quoi penses-tu?"

(What are you thinking about?)

REJECTION TRAINS DESIRE TO DIE

Dear Americans,

You can't constantly reject someone—roll away, say "not tonight," turn intimacy into a cold shoulder—and then be shocked when they stop trying. Repetition is powerful: It teaches even passion to sit, stay, and disappear. A partner who has been trained to expect rejection won't keep reaching out; they'll stop desiring altogether. In France, we know desire is fragile. It grows with encouragement, dies with dismissal. If you close the door a hundred times, don't be surprised when no one knocks anymore.

Comme on dit en France:
On n'arrose pas une fleur pour la voir faner.

As we say in France:
You don't water a flower just to watch it wilt.

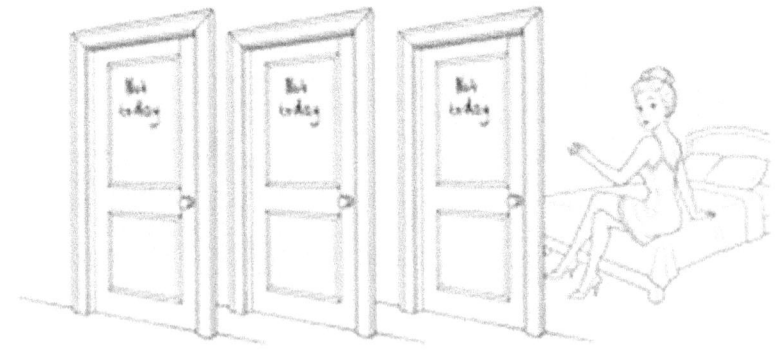

"À quoi penses-tu?"
(What are you thinking about?)

ADULTERY DOESN'T JUST END A MARRIAGE. IT ENDS EVERYTHING.

Dear Americans,

Cheating isn't an accident—it's a decision. Sleep with your best friend's wife, and you don't just betray your partner—you burn three bridges at once. Your marriage dies. His marriage dies. The friendship dies. One reckless night can kill a lifetime of trust. Call it ADHD, call it impulse, call it anything you want—it's still sabotage. In France, we know desire is fire: If you can't control where you strike the match, don't be shocked when the whole house burns down.

Comme on dit en France:
Celui qui trahit au lit détruit tout autour.

As we say in France:
He who betrays in bed destroys everything around him.

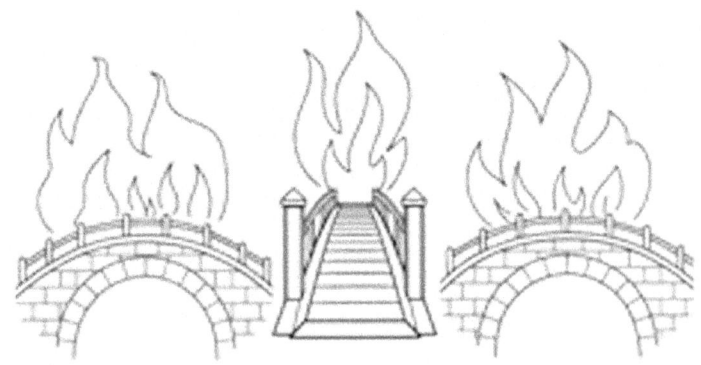

"À quoi penses-tu?"

(What are you thinking about?)

WHEN LOVE LANGUAGES MEET NARCISSISM, IT'S A TRAP

Dear Americans,

Love languages only work when there is love. With a narcissist, they become weapons. Acts of service? Taken for granted. Words of affirmation? Twisted into supply. Gifts? Demanded, never reciprocated. Touch? Only when it feeds their ego. A narcissist doesn't translate love—they exploit it. The more you give, the emptier you feel, because their hunger is bottomless. In France, we say, languages are for communication, not manipulation. With a narcissist, there's no dialogue—only monologue. And intimacy dies in that silence.

Comme on dit en France:
On ne parle pas d'amour avec un mur.

As we say in France:
You can't speak love to a wall.

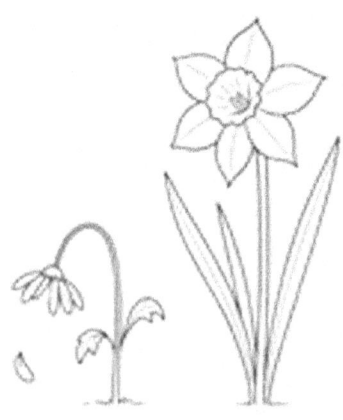

"À quoi penses-tu?"
(What are you thinking about?)

ORGASMS AREN'T THE GOAL. PRESENCE IS.

Dear Americans,

You think sex is fixed by chasing the orgasm, but intimacy is not an engine—it's a barometer. For many women, climax is not the proof of passion; the quality of the journey is. She may feel more frustrated after a shallow orgasm than after a long plateau of real presence. What defines a lover is not the fireworks but the warmth before and after. Don't chase results—create connection. That's what lasts.

Comme on dit en France:
Un orgasme ne prouve rien, mais la tendresse prouve tout.

As we say in France:
An orgasm proves nothing, but tenderness proves everything.

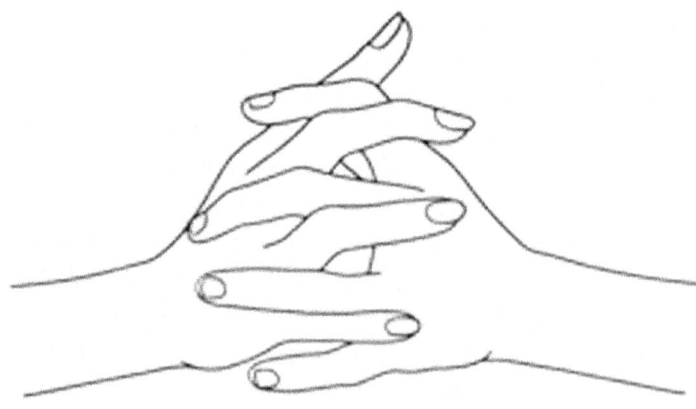

"À quoi penses-tu?"

(What are you thinking about?)

BRING CURIOSITY BACK TO THE BEDROOM

Dear Americans,

Routine kills what curiosity once kept alive. You stop asking her what she misses, what she dreams about, and then wonder why desire fades. In France, we know curiosity is not interrogation—it's invitation. When you stay curious about her soul, her body follows. Marriages don't die from too much familiarity; they die from too little wonder. Lovers who ask keep learning; lovers who stop drift into silence.

Comme on dit en France:
La curiosité rallume ce que l'habitude a éteint.

As we say in France:
Curiosity reignites what routine extinguished.

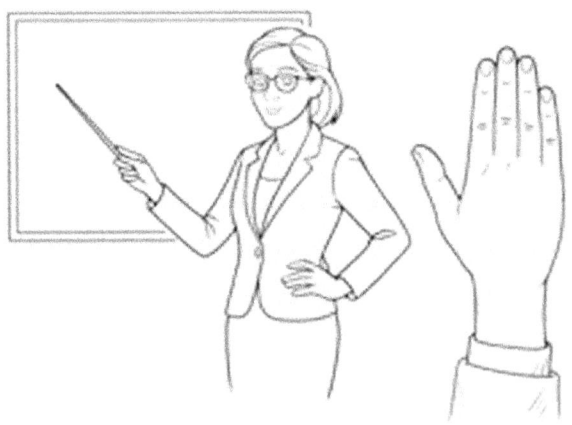

"À quoi penses-tu?"
(What are you thinking about?)

ABSENCE OF SEX
IS RARELY JUST ABOUT SEX

Dear Americans,

You think a sexless marriage is fixed by scheduling more sex. Non. Sexlessness is rarely the disease—it's the symptom. Exhaustion, resentment, unspoken anger, loneliness: These starve intimacy before the bedroom even sees it. You can't repair the bed until you repair the heart. Heal the silence, the neglect, the lack of gratitude—and then touch will return.

Comme on dit en France:
Réparer le lit commence par réparer le cœur.

As we say in France:
Fixing the bed starts with fixing the heart.

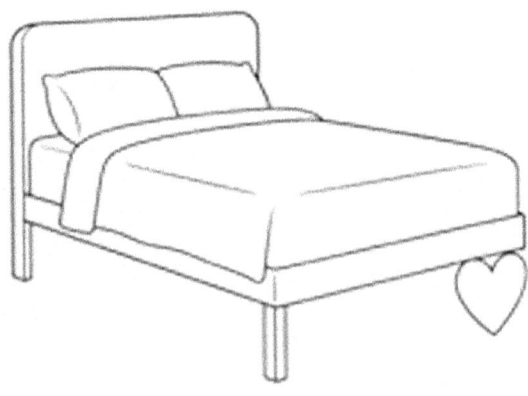

"À quoi penses-tu?"

(What are you thinking about?)

DON'T LET SILENCE WIN

Dear Americans,

Every night you say nothing, distance wins. Intimacy doesn't die in arguments—it dies in shrugs and silences. Don't wait for the perfect talk. Whisper something. Reach for her hand. Even clumsy words are proof you still care. In France, we know silence in bed is not romantic, it's a funeral. Don't let it become the third partner between you.

Comme on dit en France:
L'intimité meurt quand le silence s'installe.

As we say in France:
Intimacy dies when silence settles in.

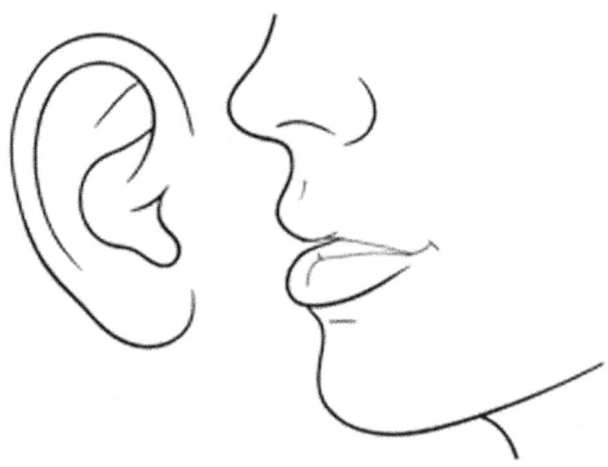

"À quoi penses-tu?"

(What are you thinking about?)

PRESENT IN THE HOUSE, ABSENT IN THE HEART

Dear Americans,

He's in the house. His shoes by the door, his body in the bed. But his heart? Absent. A woman doesn't need a room-mate who pays the mortgage—she needs presence. Walls don't make her feel loved; warmth does. In France, we know lying next to her every night means nothing if your heart is miles away.

Comme on dit en France:
Tu peux être à côté d'elle chaque nuit,
et pourtant si loin de son cœur.

As we say in France:
You can lie beside her every night and
still be miles from her heart.

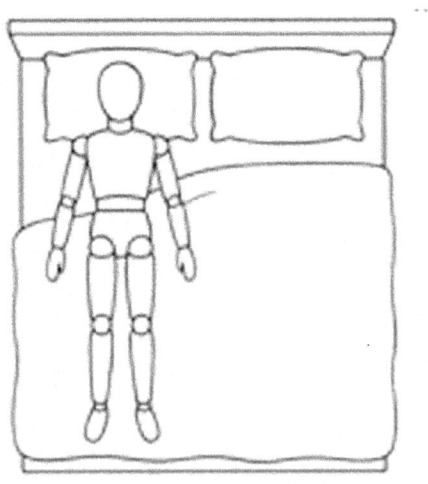

"À quoi penses-tu?"

(What are you thinking about?)

FROM PARTNER TO ROOMMATE

Dear Americans,

You began as lovers, hungry for each other. Now you are co-managers of errands. Groceries. School runs. Repairs. The romance is replaced with routines, the passion with paperwork. She didn't marry a housemate—she married a man who once desired her. In France, we know love can survive many storms but not being reduced to logistics.

Comme on dit en France:
L'amour n'a jamais signé un bail.

As we say in France:
Love never signed a lease.

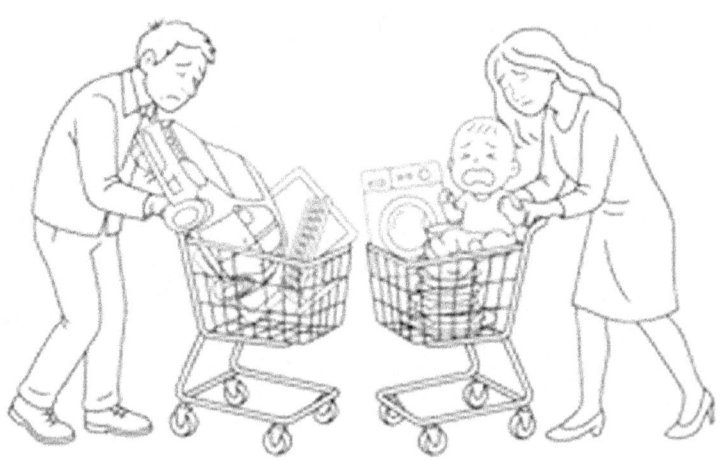

"À quoi penses-tu?"

(What are you thinking about?)

SHE MISSES THE MAN WHO FLIRTED

Dear Americans,

Once upon a time, you sent cheeky texts and made her blush while cooking. Now it's "Pick up milk." Roses are not the point—desire is. She doesn't need clichés; she needs proof she still stirs you. In France, we don't retire from flirting—we refine it. Flirtation is not childish; it is fuel.

Comme on dit en France:
Un petit clin d'œil vaut plus qu'un gros bouquet.

As we say in France:
One cheeky wink is worth more than a giant bouquet.

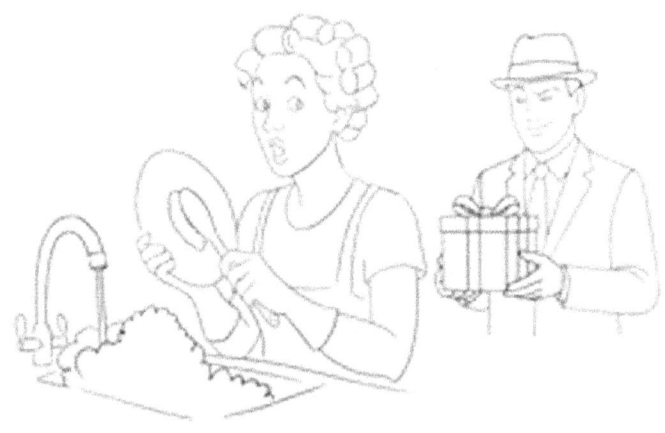

"À quoi penses-tu?"
(What are you thinking about?)

GRUNTS ARE NOT COMMUNICATION

Dear Americans,

"He used to ask about my dreams. Now he just nods between bites." Grunts and sighs aren't conversation. A woman doesn't starve from lack of food—she starves from lack of words. Intimacy begins with attention, not silence. In France, we don't believe in love that sounds like indigestion.

Comme on dit en France:
Un soupir ne remplace pas une phrase d'amour.

As we say in France:
A grunt can't replace a phrase of love.

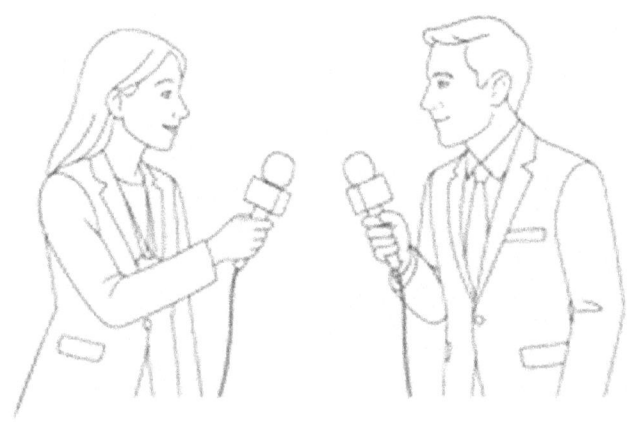

"À quoi penses-tu?"

(What are you thinking about?)

SHE TALKS ABOUT BILLS...
NOT ABOUT "US"

Dear Americans,

The budget is balanced. The fence painted. The fridge stocked. But when was the last time you talked about "us"? Some marriages don't collapse in storms—they die quietly in spreadsheets. She doesn't want another accountant; she wants a lover. In France, we know you can't make love with a shopping list.

Comme on dit en France:
On ne fait pas l'amour avec une liste de courses.

As we say in France:
You can't make love with a shopping list.

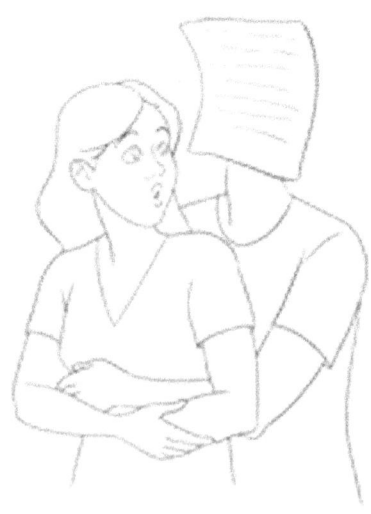

"À quoi penses-tu?"

(What are you thinking about?)

A GOOD MAN ISN'T ALWAYS AN ENGAGED ONE

Dear Americans,

He's loyal. Faithful. Hardworking. On paper, perfect. But love isn't lived on paper—it's lived in presence. Many women don't leave because of betrayal; they leave because of emptiness. A man who never cheats but never shows up emotionally is still abandoning her. She doesn't need protection—she needs connection. In France, we know passion is not proven by fidelity alone, but by daily devotion.

Comme on dit en France:
Elle n'a pas besoin d'un garde du corps, mais d'un cœur présent.

As we say in France:
She doesn't need a bodyguard—she needs a present heart.

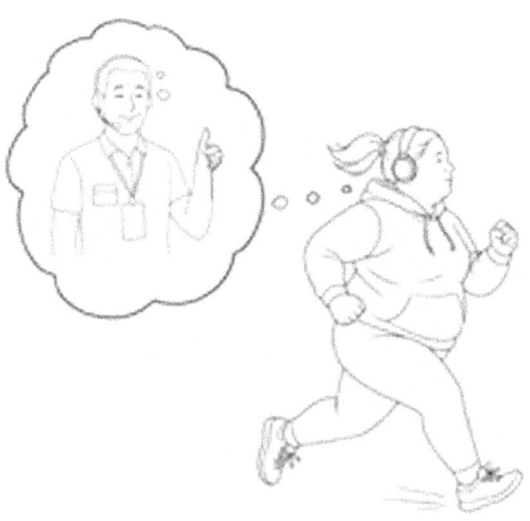

"À quoi penses-tu?"
(What are you thinking about?)

SEE WHAT SHE CARRIES

Dear Americans,

Her purse is not just keys and lipstick—it's your moods, her mother's aging, the pediatrician's number, and the endless lists that keep your world spinning. She looks polished, but behind the smile is fatigue. She doesn't want rescue—she wants recognition. Ask what no one else asks: "What are you carrying that no one sees?" That answer is intimacy itself.

Comme on dit en France:
Elle porte plus que son sac à main.

As we say in France:
She's carrying more than just her purse.

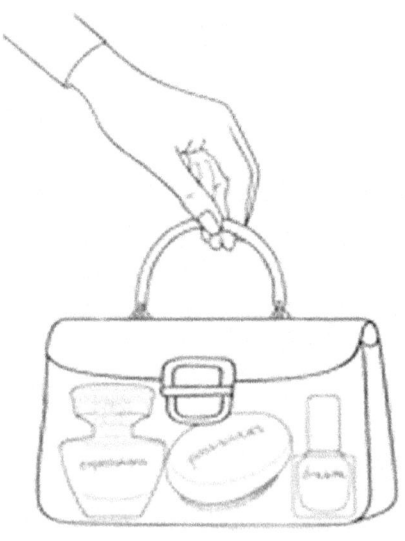

"À quoi penses-tu?"

(What are you thinking about?)

ASK WHERE SHE FEELS OVERWHELMED

Dear Americans,

Seduction begins before the bedroom. Don't only ask what she wants in bed—ask where life crushes her spirit, where her days drain her. Listen, not to fix, but to hold. The sexiest phrase isn't "You're hot." It's: "Tell me where it hurts." Attention is intimacy. When a woman feels heard in her struggles, her desire for you grows, because safety is erotic.

Comme on dit en France:
L'émotion entendue devient une émotion partagée.

As we say in France:
Eotion heard becomes emotion shared.

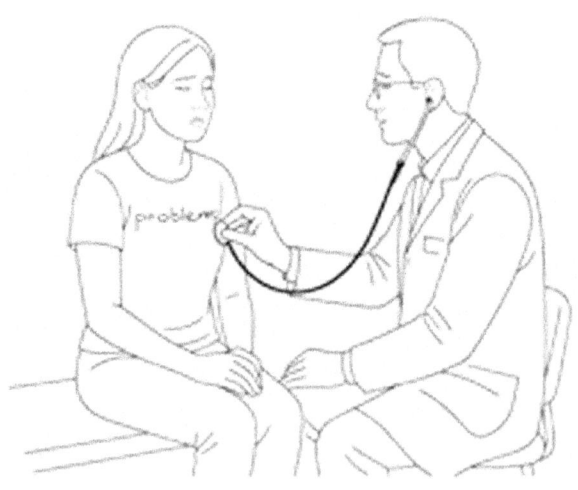

"À quoi penses-tu?"

(What are you thinking about?)

SHARE THE LOAD

Dear Americans,

Romance isn't only in Paris—it's in the dishwasher. In wiping the counter before she asks. In carrying backpacks while she breathes. Love isn't "helping"—it's partnering. You don't earn applause for pulling your weight. You earn intimacy by proving she's not alone. When she sees you shoulder life with her, she relaxes. And when she relaxes, she desires. Equality is not politics—it's foreplay.

Comme on dit en France… l'amour
commence avec le lave-vaisselle.

As we say in France… love begins with the dishwasher.

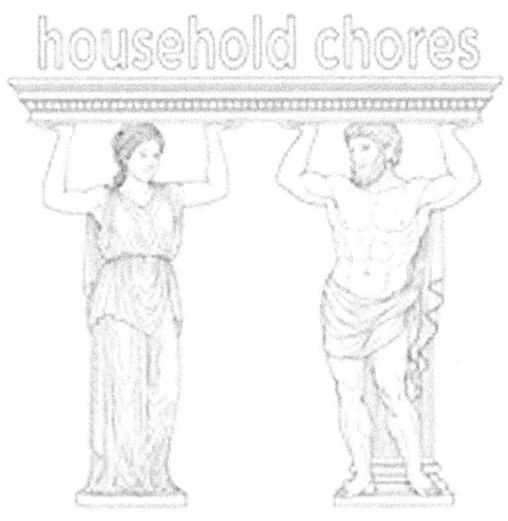

"À quoi penses-tu?"

(What are you thinking about?)

DON'T JUST SAY "YOU'RE AMAZING." PROVE IT

Dear Americans,

Flattery without action is cheap. Don't just call her strong—give her permission to rest. Don't just say she's beautiful—handle the bedtime routine so she can breathe. Words flatter, but gestures sustain. True love doesn't need speeches; it needs sacrifice. If your admiration doesn't lighten her burden, it's just noise. Lift what exhausts her, not with duty, but devotion.

Comme on dit en France:
Les mots n'essuient pas les larmes, les gestes oui.

As we say in France:
Words don't wipe tears—actions do.

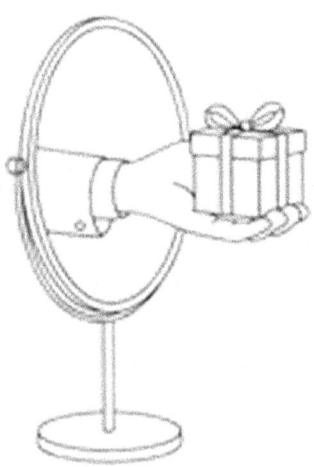

244

"À quoi penses-tu?"
(What are you thinking about?)

TRUTH #123

COMPLIMENT HER SPIRIT, NOT JUST HER LOOKS

Dear Americans,

Compliments that matter are not about waistlines. Tell her she's radiant when she speaks her truth. Admire her courage, her wisdom, her grace in chaos. She doesn't want to feel only pretty—she wants to feel alive, seen beyond the mirror. Desire doesn't begin with "sexy body." It begins with reverence for the fire within. When you praise her soul, her body responds with gratitude.

Comme on dit en France:
La beauté du cœur allume celle du corps.

As we say in France:
The beauty of the heart ignites that of the body.

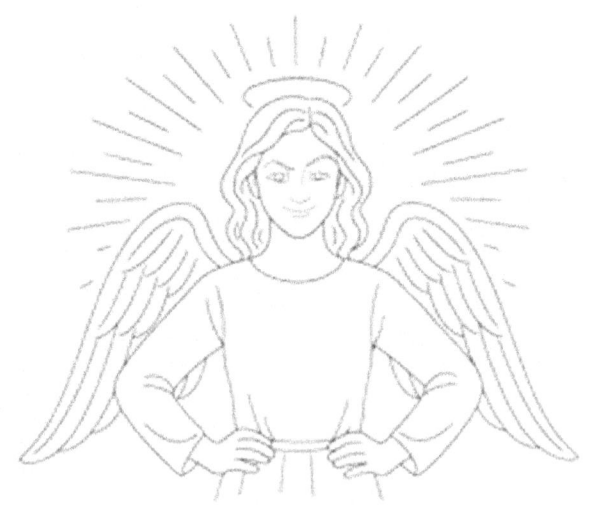

"À quoi penses-tu?"
(What are you thinking about?)

TRUTH #124

MAKE SPACE FOR HER TO BE SOFT AGAIN

Dear Americans,

Her armor is not rebellion—it's survival. Each day, she straps it on because the world demands it. Deadlines, judgments, responsibilities—they harden her. But beneath the toughness is softness waiting to breathe. She longs for a space where she doesn't have to fight, where tenderness is safe. Your role is not to strip away her defenses but to create safety for her to lay them down. That's when you'll meet her true heart.

Comme on dit en France:
Elle enlèvera l'armure si elle se sent en sécurité.

As we say in France:
She'll remove the armor if she feels safe.

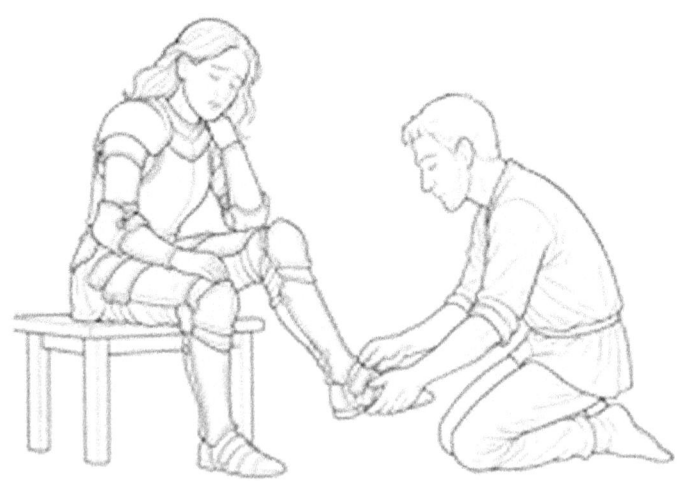

"À quoi penses-tu?"
(What are you thinking about?)

THE GLOW YOU MISS
IS BURIED UNDER TASKS

Dear Americans,

That sparkle in her eyes? The laugh that lit up the room? It's not gone—it's buried. Buried under laundry piles, deadlines, invisible labor. Romance hasn't vanished; it's suffocated by exhaustion. Don't ask her to "come back." She will return when her load is lighter. If you want her glow again, ease her burdens. Carry some weight. Help her breathe. Rest brings radiance—and radiance restores desire.

Comme on dit en France:
Elle ne manque pas de lumière, elle manque de repos.

As we say in France:
She's not missing light—she's missing rest.

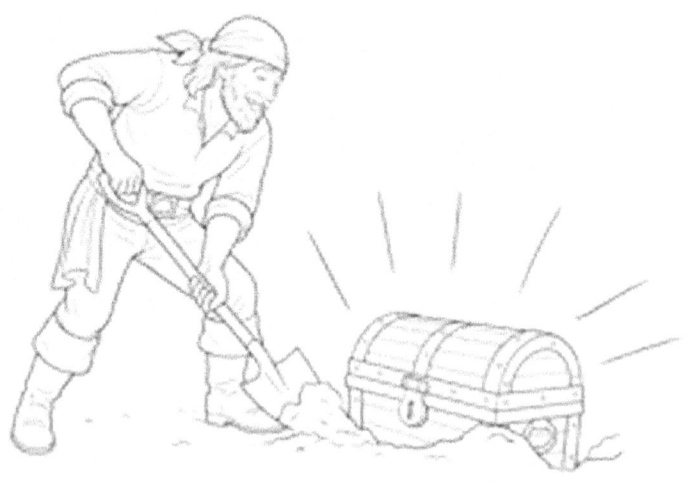

"À quoi penses-tu?"

(What are you thinking about?)

DON'T TAKE IT PERSONALLY. TAKE IT SERIOUSLY

Dear Americans,

Her silence is not rejection. Her distance is not about you—it's her body collapsing under pressure. She's not avoiding your love; she's drowning in demands. Don't get defensive. Don't sulk. Take it seriously—her exhaustion is a plea for care. Ask what she needs and listen with humility. When she feels supported instead of blamed, closeness returns like a tide.

Comme on dit en France:
Ce qu'elle fuit, ce n'est pas toi, c'est le poids.

As we say in France:
It's not you she's avoiding—it's the weight.

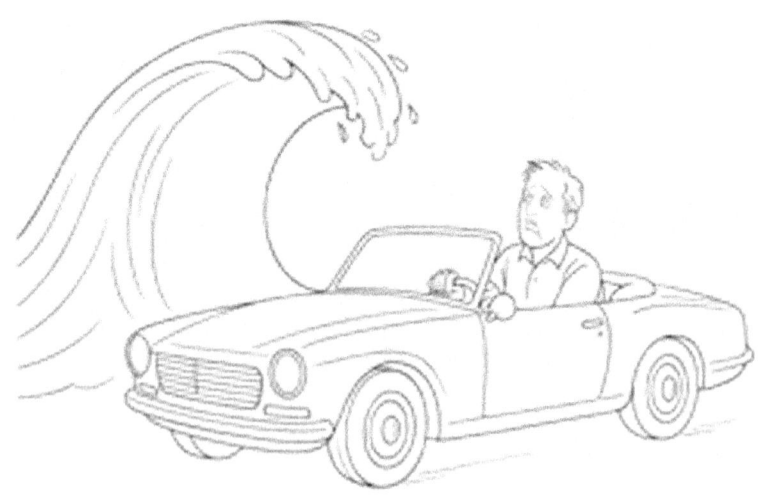

"À quoi penses-tu?"

(What are you thinking about?)

TRUTH #127

DESIRE IS BORN WHEN THE LOAD IS LIGHTENED

Dear Americans,

Passion cannot be demanded from a woman buried in stress. Desire doesn't bloom in pressure; it blooms in peace. She doesn't need more seduction; she needs support. Wash the dishes. Pay the bill. Take something off her mind—not as a transaction but as devotion. When she feels free, her sensuality breathes again. Passion isn't forced—it's unlocked.

Comme on dit en France:
Le désir respire dans l'espace qu'on lui laisse.

As we say in France:
Desire breathes in the space it's given.

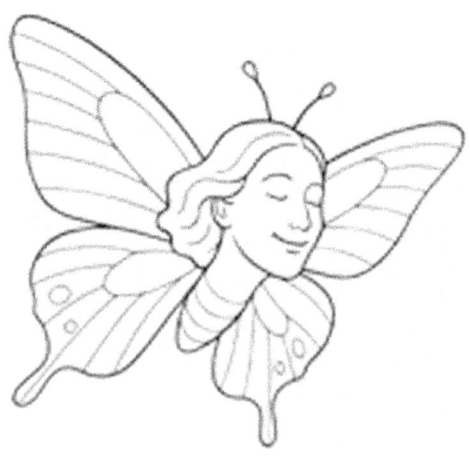

"À quoi penses-tu?"
(What are you thinking about?)

BRING BACK THE GAZE

Dear Americans,

Every woman remembers how her man once looked at her—hungry, enchanted, undone. Over time, the gaze fades, replaced by shrugs, glances, and screens. She hasn't lost her beauty—you've lost your eyes. Desire is not about lingerie or Botox—it's about being seen. Look again. She's still your masterpiece. When a man forgets to look, love forgets to live. If you want passion back, begin with your gaze—it is the first flame of intimacy, and often the last to die when neglected.

Comme on dit en France:
Elle veut ton regard, pas juste ta présence.

As we say in France:
She wants your gaze, not just your presence.

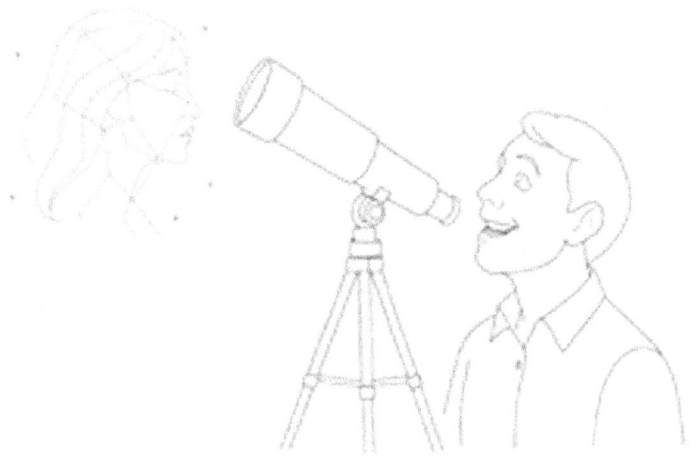

"À quoi penses-tu?"

(What are you thinking about?)

LOVE NEEDS MAINTENANCE, TOO

Dear Americans,

You service your car. You trim the lawn. You update your phone. But when was the last time you tuned your marriage? Love is not a "set it and forget it" machine—it's a living garden. Without care, it rusts, it withers, it collapses. A woman doesn't want grand gestures once a year—she wants steady devotion every day. Preventive maintenance saves engines; it also saves marriages. Romance requires attention, and attention is the oil that keeps love from breaking down. Don't neglect it and wonder why the engine stalls.

Comme on dit en France:
Le cœur a besoin d'entretien, sinon il rouille.

As we say in France:
The heart needs maintenance—or it rusts.

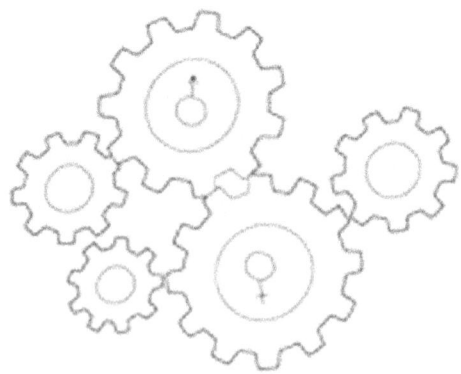

"À quoi penses-tu?"

(What are you thinking about?)

TRUTH #130

SHE DOESN'T WANT A ROOMMATE—SHE WANTS A CO-CONSPIRATOR

Dear Americans,

Life already drowns us in chores, budgets, and responsibilities. She doesn't want another housemate who pays bills—she wants a partner who plays. Someone who laughs with her, who plots escapes, who turns the ordinary into adventure. Desire thrives not in spreadsheets but in conspiracies—inside jokes, little rebellions, secrets only the two of you share. A roommate shares space; a co-conspirator shares passion. Which one do you want to be?

Comme on dit en France:
Elle ne veut pas de colocataire, mais un complice.

As we say in France:
She doesn't want a roommate—she wants a partner in crime.

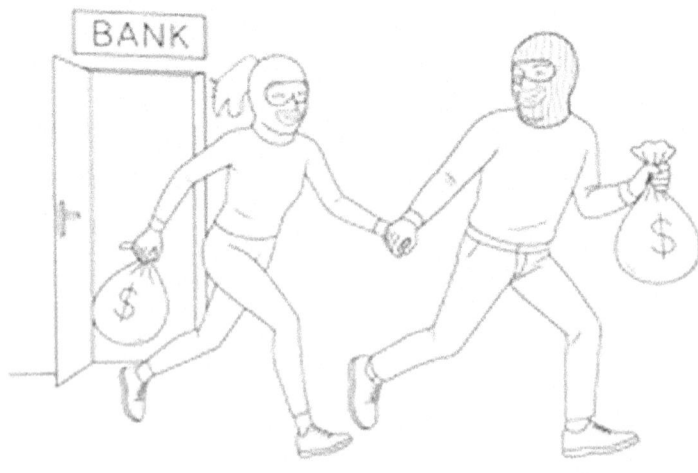

"À quoi penses-tu?"

(What are you thinking about?)

MARRIAGE IS NOT A FINISH LINE

Dear Americans,

Marriage isn't the grand finale—it's the opening act. Too many couples treat the wedding as the destination instead of the doorway. The vows are not medals; they're invitations to keep showing up. Romance, laughter, and seduction don't retire with rings—they must be practiced daily. Love is not a trophy gathering dust—it's a ritual that breathes only if you feed it. Don't treat "I do" as the ending credits; treat it as the first line of the script.

Comme on dit en France:
Le "oui" n'est pas la fin, c'est le commencement.

As we say in France:
"I do" isn't the end—it's the beginning.

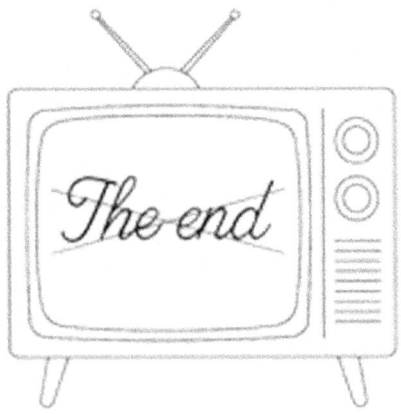

"À quoi penses-tu?"

(What are you thinking about?)

THE CHASE SHOULD NEVER END

Dear Americans,

Remember the thrill of pursuit? The butterflies? The spark? That energy didn't die—it was abandoned. Love withers when curiosity fades and routine replace romance. Women still want to be courted—not with roses every day, but with attention, surprise, and effort. The chase never ends, because desire dies when it feels taken for granted. A teasing text, a whispered "I still want you," a kiss in the kitchen—that's pursuit in real time.

Comme on dit en France:
L'amour s'endort quand la chasse s'arrête.

As we say in France:
Love falls asleep when the chase ends.

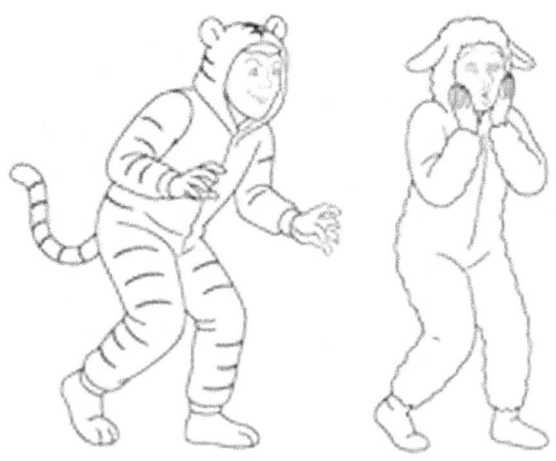

"À quoi penses-tu?"

(What are you thinking about?)

SHE'S NOT A TROPHY

Dear Americans,

A woman doesn't want to be displayed, admired, but untouched. She doesn't want duty disguised as desire. She craves passion, intimacy, presence—the kind that proves she's still fire, not furniture. A trophy is static, lifeless, symbolic. A woman is living heat, craving fuel. If you stop feeding the flame, don't be surprised when the fire dies. Keep seeing her, touching her, choosing her—she is not for decoration, she is for devotion.

Comme on dit en France:
Une femme n'est pas un trophée, c'est une flamme à nourrir.

As we say in France:
A woman isn't a trophy—she's a flame to be kept alive.

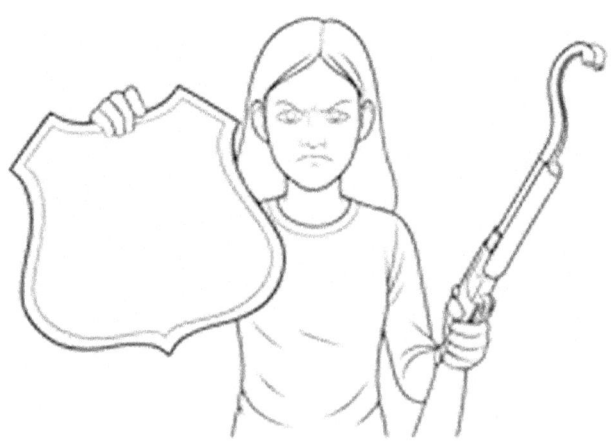

"À quoi penses-tu?"

(What are you thinking about?)

AFTER THE WEDDING, THE ATTENTION VANISHED

Dear Americans,

He planned every detail, wrote vows, swept her off her feet—until the "after." Too many men believe the win is the wedding, when the real work begins once the applause fades. Attention, romance, and seduction matter more when life gets heavy, not less. She doesn't want a man who conquered her once; she wants one who keeps choosing her daily. The honeymoon phase is not supposed to die—it's supposed to evolve.

Comme on dit en France:
Ce n'est pas le mariage qui compte, c'est ce que tu en fais après.

As we say in France:
The wedding isn't what matters—it's what you do after.

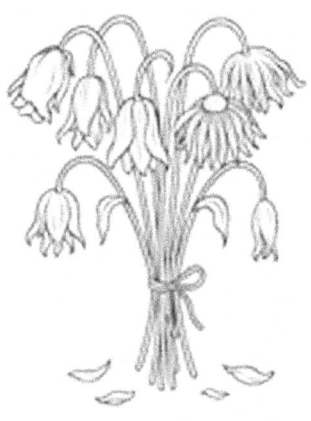

268

"À quoi penses-tu?"
(What are you thinking about?)

TRUTH #135

YOU STOPPED NOTICING HER

Dear Americans,

Desire doesn't die overnight—it dies in silence. It dies in the ignored glance, the overlooked detail, the absence of "You're beautiful." A woman fades not from age, but from invisibility. She won't always leave in anger—she leaves when she feels unseen in her own home. Notice her dress. Notice her laugh. Notice her presence—or risk her absence. The easiest way to lose her is to stop looking.

Comme on dit en France:
Ignorer, c'est commencer à perdre.

As we say in France:
Ignoring is the first step to losing.

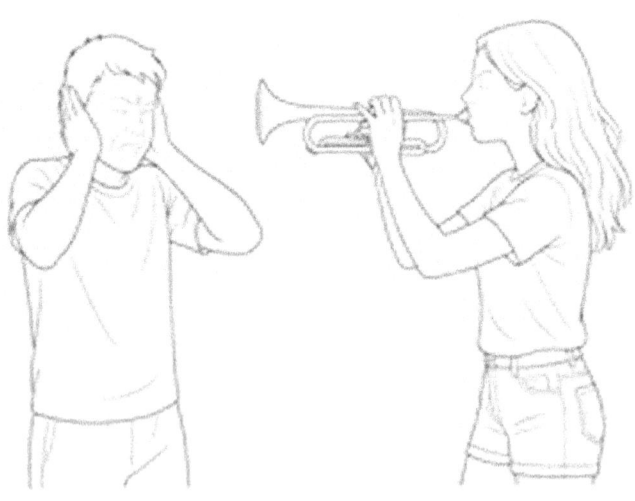

"À quoi penses-tu?"

(What are you thinking about?)

LOVE IS NOT GYMNASTICS

Dear Americans,

How to make love well? It isn't hidden in acrobatic positions or borrowed tricks from a magazine. The deepest orgasms don't come from circus acts; they come from connection. When two partners feel safe, adored, and truly loved, the body follows naturally. Passion grows not in contortions but in devotion. A look, a touch, a word of presence can be more explosive than fifteen rehearsed moves. Sex isn't about performance—it's about communion. Love is the greatest aphrodisiac of all.

Comme on dit en France:
Le vrai orgasme naît de la connexion, pas de la gymnastique.

As we say in France:
The real orgasm comes from connection, not gymnastics.

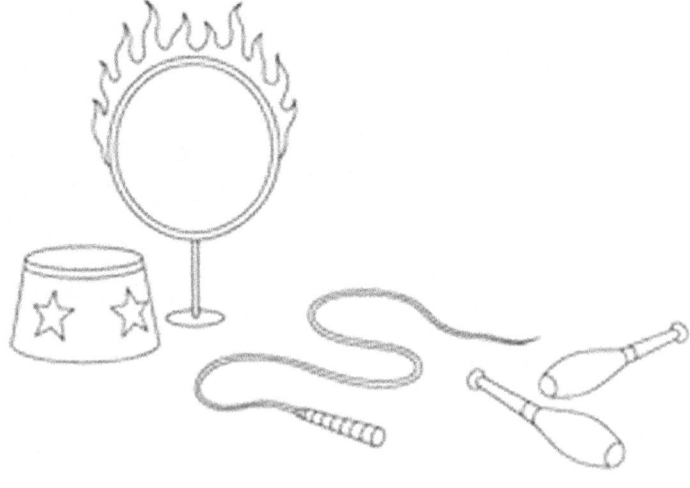

"À quoi penses-tu?"
(What are you thinking about?)

ORAL SEX IS NOT A ONE-WAY STREET

Dear Americans,

Too many men expect to receive but forget to give. Desire dies in imbalance. A woman's pleasure is not a bonus—it is the foundation of intimacy. Neglecting her is not only selfish; it's shortsighted. In France, we know generosity in bed feeds devotion outside of it. When you kneel to worship her body, you're not losing power—you're gaining loyalty, tenderness, and fire. Reciprocity is not an option; it is the oxygen of passion. If you want her to crave you, then first, make her feel consumed by you.

Comme on dit en France:
Le désir se nourrit de réciprocité.

As we say in France:
Desire feeds on reciprocity.

"À quoi penses-tu?"
(What are you thinking about?)

FOUR SIGNS HE'S TRULY IN LOVE

Dear Americans,

Sex shows what words hide. A man who is truly in love reveals it between the sheets. First, his gaze—he looks into your soul, not just your body. Second, his unconscious gestures—touches that comfort, not just consume. Third, his gentleness after love—because real passion doesn't roll away, it stays and holds. Fourth, the details: how he notices your sighs, your smile, your stillness. Intimacy is the unconscious speaking aloud. If you want to know if he loves you, don't listen to his promises—watch his presence in bed.

Comme on dit en France:
L'amour se voit dans les détails.

As we say in France:
Love is seen in the details.

"À quoi penses-tu?"

(What are you thinking about?)

DIVORCE AFTER SIXTY IS NOT THE END—IT'S THE REBIRTH

Dear Americans,

In the last thirty years, divorces after sixty have doubled—and in most cases, it's women walking away. Why? Because longer lives, better health, and emancipation have given them choices their mothers never had. Many don't see divorce as an ending, but as a second youth. Dating apps are full of silver-haired rebels daring to begin again. Marriages over sixty have risen 18 percent, proving desire doesn't retire. Don't bury your body before the grave. Celebrate it until the last day—because passion isn't just for the young, it's for the alive.

Comme on dit en France:
Le désir n'a pas d'âge.

As we say in France:
Desire has no age.

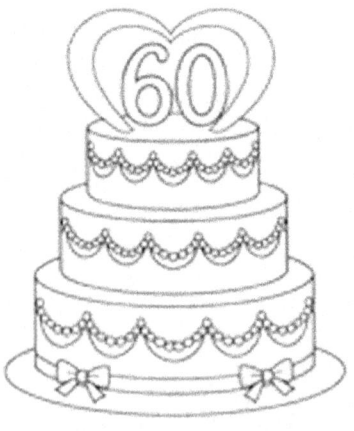

"À quoi penses-tu?"

(What are you thinking about?)

MARRIAGE ISN'T A FAIRY TALE— IT'S A BATTLEFIELD WITH KISSES

Dear Americans,

Let's be real: Marriage isn't all date nights and Netflix cuddles. It's messy. Emotional. Sometimes painfully lonely, even when you share the same bed. Love isn't destroyed by shouting matches—it's worn down by silence, exhaustion, and routine. But the couples who survive are not the ones who avoid the mess; they're the ones who keep reaching through it. Marriage is less about perfection and more about persistence—the art of choosing each other even on the ugliest days.

Comme on dit en France:
Le vrai amour porte des cicatrices.

As we say in France:
Real love wears scars.

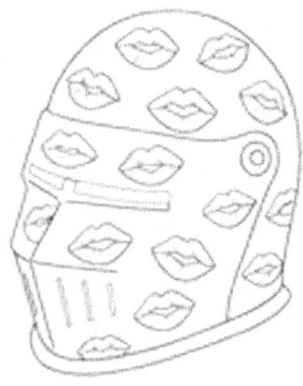

"À quoi penses-tu?"

(What are you thinking about?)

LOVE ISN'T A FEELING— IT'S A DISCIPLINE

Dear Americans,

Butterflies do not sustain marriage; daily choices do. Real love is the act of showing up, especially when it's inconvenient. You can't neglect communication, abandon tenderness, and still call it love. When you vowed to love, you didn't promise comfort—you promised commitment. The true test of character isn't how you behave when love feels easy, but how you act when it demands effort. When you stop nurturing the person who believed in you, you don't lose a partner—you reveal your immaturity.

Comme on dit en France:
L'amour se prouve quand c'est difficile, pas quand c'est facile.

As we say in France:
Love is proven when it's hard, not when it's easy.

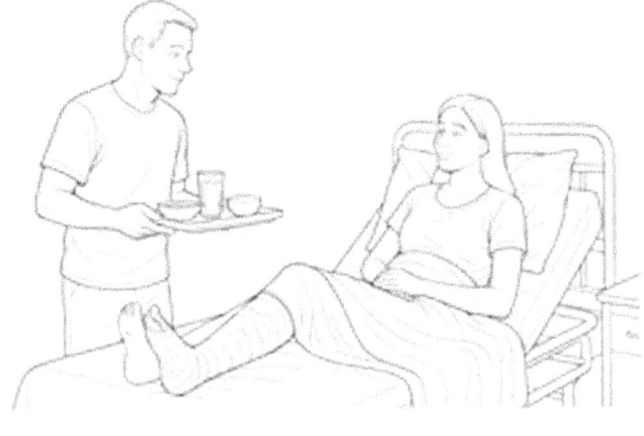

"À quoi penses-tu?"

(What are you thinking about?)

Marriage Isn't for the Faint of Heart

Dear Americans,

Marriage is not a fairy tale—it's a battlefield of patience, honesty, and endurance. In a world where divorce is celebrated like freedom and violence lurks behind wedding photos, choose wisely. Remember your vows. Examine your motives. Are you partners or just cohabitants waiting for the clock to strike eighteen on your children's birthdays? Marriage today demands courage—to stay, to communicate, to grow, and sometimes to walk away with dignity. Love isn't soft. It's sacred labor.

Comme on dit en France:
Le mariage n'est pas pour les faibles,
mais pour les courageux du cœur.

As we say in France:
Marriage isn't for the weak, but for the brave of heart.

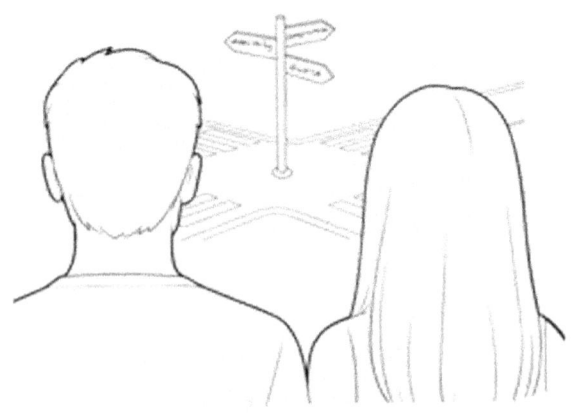

284

"À quoi penses-tu?"

(What are you thinking about?)

YOU CAN'T MAKE A MAN FALL IN LOVE

Dear Americans,

Love isn't a strategy—it's chemistry. You can't "make" a man fall in love any more than you can force the sun to rise faster. If the connection is real, it reveals itself in gestures, not games. If he doesn't prove it through consistency, tenderness, and presence, then he's not in love—he's just entertained. Feminine charm isn't manipulation; it's authenticity. A woman's power isn't in convincing—it's in being. The body never lies, and real attraction needs no script.

Comme on dit en France:
L'amour ne se fabrique pas, il se reconnaît.

As we say in France:
Love isn't made—it's recognized.

"À quoi penses-tu?"

(What are you thinking about?)

FINANCIAL INFIDELITY KILLS INTIMACY

Dear Americans,

You talk about love, dreams, even trauma—but not money. Yet money is one of the most intimate subjects of all. When one partner hides expenses, debts, or earnings, it's not just deception—it's domination. Financial infidelity creates silent hierarchies: one gives, the other begs; one controls, the other obeys. And where there's secrecy, desire suffocates. You can't make love freely when one person holds the receipts of power. Transparency isn't about accounting—it's about trust.

Comme on dit en France:
Le secret tue le désir plus vite que la pauvreté.

As we say in France:
Secrecy kills desire faster than poverty.

"À quoi penses-tu?"

(What are you thinking about?)

FINANCIAL CONTROL IS MODERN VIOLENCE

Dear Americans,

When one partner controls the money, they control the other's freedom. That's not love—it's domination. Financial infidelity may not leave bruises, but it leaves fear, silence, and dependence. It's a quiet form of domestic violence, wrapped in budgets and bank accounts. The "breadwinner" who dictates every decision isn't a provider—he's a warden. True partnership means shared power, not permission. Economic independence is protection—it's dignity. Until equality becomes law, let it begin at home.

Comme on dit en France:
Celui qui contrôle l'argent contrôle la liberté.

As we say in France:
Whoever controls the money controls the freedom.

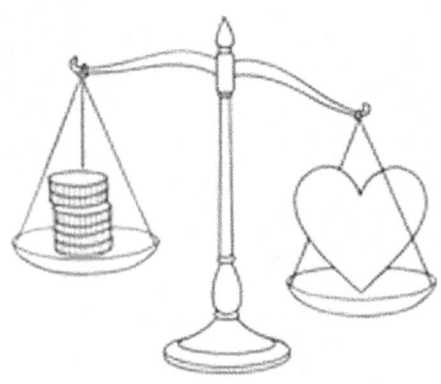

"À quoi penses-tu?"

(What are you thinking about?)

DRY WOOD DOESN'T CATCH FIRE

Dear Americans,

You can't light a blaze with wet wood. When your partner is soaked in stress, resentment, or exhaustion, no technique will make her burn. Desire needs oxygen—peace, safety, and time to breathe. Ease her load, protect her rest, and calm her storms. Then you'll watch sparks turn to flames. Passion doesn't respond to pressure; it responds to presence. Dry the wood first—then the fire will come alive.

Comme on dit en France:
Le feu de l'amour a besoin d'air.

As we say in France:
Love's fire needs air.

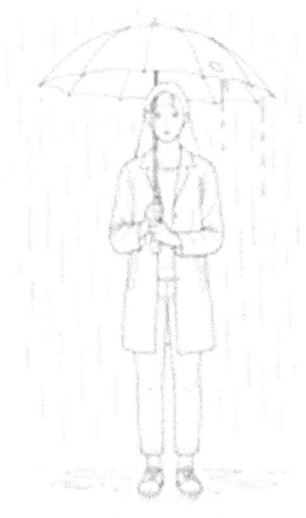

"À quoi penses-tu?"
(What are you thinking about?)

BE THE MAN OTHERS RESPECT—
AND SHE CHOOSES

Dear Americans,

A woman's desire sharpens when she sees her man admired. It's not vanity—it's instinct. When you carry yourself with confidence, kindness, and quiet power, she sees what others see—and it reignites her pride to be yours. Be magnetic, not boastful. Presence, not posing. She doesn't need a hero with muscles; she needs a man with gravity. Enter a room with grace, and she'll want the encore in private.

Comme on dit en France:
Le charme se voit avant de se toucher.

As we say in France:
Charm is seen before it's touched.

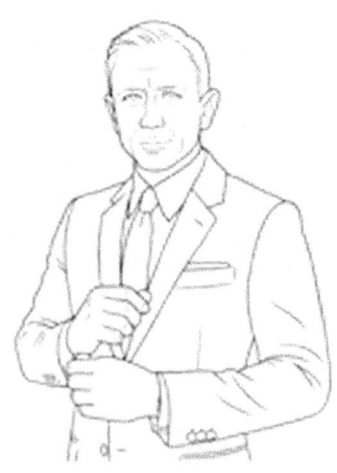

"À quoi penses-tu?"

(What are you thinking about?)

SEDUCE MIND + BODY OR SEDUCE NO ONE

Dear Americans,

If you touch her body but ignore her soul, she'll give you skin, not surrender. Ask, listen, remember—flirt with her intelligence, not just her lips. The greatest lovers seduce thought before thigh. Attention is foreplay; curiosity is arousal. When a woman feels seen beyond her surface, her body becomes an open letter. Don't just perform—connect.

Comme on dit en France:
Sans tête, le cœur se ferme.

As we say in France:
Without the mind, the heart closes.

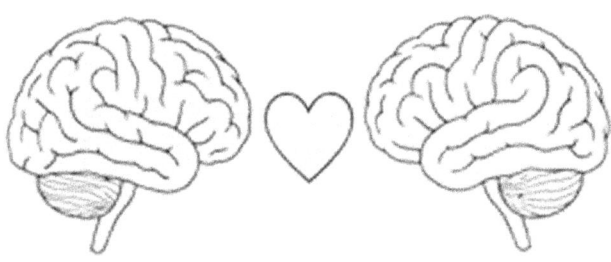

"À quoi penses-tu?"

(What are you thinking about?)

TRUTH #149

BUILD THE EROTIC SAFE ROOM

Dear Americans,

Judgment kills desire faster than age ever could. Create a space where her fantasies can breathe—where no part of her feels too much or too strange. When she feels safe, she stops censoring her pleasure. Invite her wildness and protect it fiercely. The best lovers don't command—they liberate. Safety is the gateway to audacity.

Comme on dit en France:
la sécurité allume l'audace.

As we say in France:
Safety lights boldness.

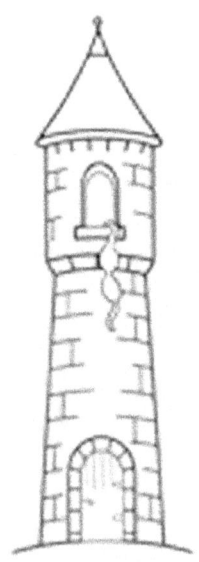

"À quoi penses-tu?"
(What are you thinking about?)

HEALTH, POSTURE, VOICE: YOUR REAL APHRODISIACS

Dear Americans,

You don't need a superhero's body to be desired. Stay healthy, smell clean, move like you mean it. Stand tall—not rigid but grounded. Your voice is your secret weapon: whisper, pause, let silence seduce. Engage all five senses—touch, taste, scent, sight, sound. Eroticism is not performance—it's presence. Learn to move with rhythm and intention, and she'll feel it before you touch her.

Comme on dit en France:
l'érotisme est une cuisine à cinq saveurs.

As we say in France:
Eroticism is a five-flavor kitchen.

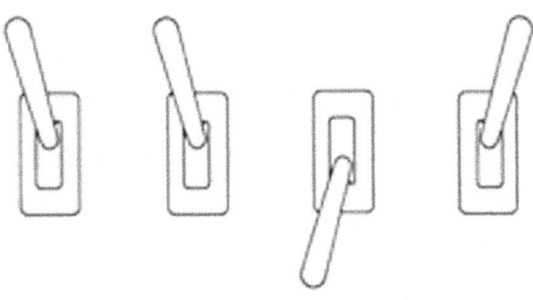

"À quoi penses-tu?"

(What are you thinking about?)

THE COMPETITION
THAT SAVES LOVE

Dear Americans,

The best relationships aren't about who wins the argument—they're about who gives more love. When both partners make each other's happiness the priority, something magical happens; ego fades, tenderness grows, and gratitude replaces resentment. The healthiest couples quietly compete—not to dominate, but to out-care, out-serve, and out-love each other. They don't keep score because both are winning. Two people who put each other first create a cycle of devotion that no storm can break.

Comme on dit en France:
Aimer, c'est rivaliser de générosité.

As we say in France:
Love is a competition in generosity.

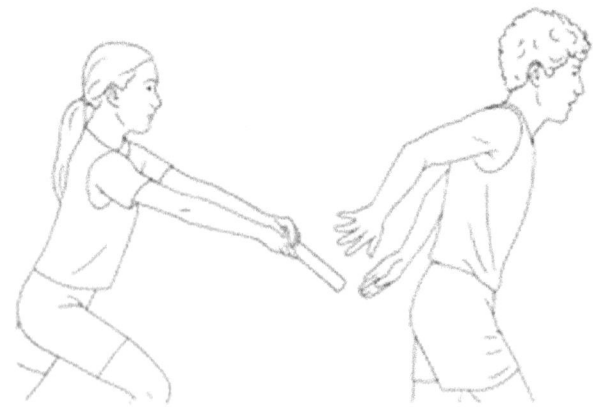

"À quoi penses-tu?"

(What are you thinking about?)

SCREENS ARE THE NEW MISTRESS

Dear Americans,

You can't build intimacy in a room lit by blue light. Phones have become the third partner in too many beds—always buzzing, always stealing presence. Once upon a time, we survived without notifications. We looked at each other, not at a glowing screen. Make your bedroom sacred again. Leave your phones charging in the kitchen and let your minds recharge together. After love, don't reach for the digital world—reach for your partner. Connection dies when the screen replaces the gaze.

Comme on dit en France:
Le vrai signal, c'est le regard.

As we say in France:
The real signal is the gaze.

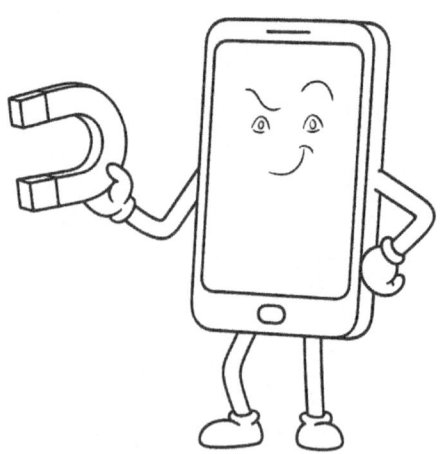

"À quoi penses-tu?"
(What are you thinking about?)

YOU CAN'T JUST SHOW UP. YOU HAVE TO PLUG IN

Dear Americans,

Proximity is not intimacy. Sitting on the same couch while scrolling Instagram doesn't make you a partner; it makes you furniture. She doesn't want a roommate; she wants a lover who plugs into her—her laugh, her silence, her chaos. In France, we say, Wi-Fi is fast, but the heart is rare. So put the phone down and tune in. If you don't, Netflix will have more of her attention than you do.

Comme on dit en France:
La connexion la plus rare, c'est celle du cœur.

As we say in France:
The rarest connection is the one from the heart.

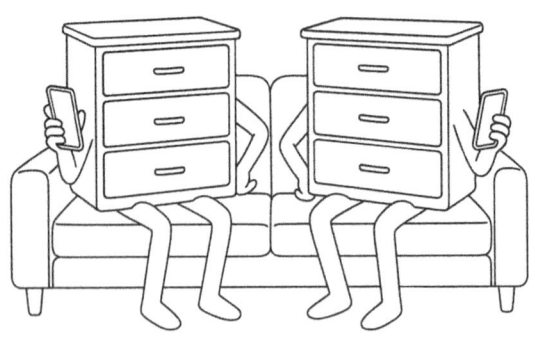

306

"À quoi penses-tu?"
(What are you thinking about?)

CONCLUSION

THE REAL REVOLUTION
STARTS AT HOME

Dear Americans,

We've dissected the sexless, the silent, the screen-addicted, and the emotionally constipated. We've explored what desire truly means—beyond hormones and hashtags. Now, let's be honest: The real revolution in America won't happen in Congress or on TikTok. It will happen in bedrooms, where two people finally decide to look at each other again instead of at a phone.

Marriage, intimacy, and pleasure aren't political. They're human. And when couples start rebuilding connection—one gaze, one touch, one honest conversation at a time—that's when the nation begins to heal.

Comme on dit en France:
La révolution commence sous les draps.

As we say in France:
Revolution begins under the sheets.

TURN OFF THE NEWS, TURN ON EACH OTHER

Dear Americans,

After the next election, half the country will sulk, and the other half will celebrate. But here's a radical idea: Instead of watching endless debates, go make love.

Turn off CNN, FOX, and every expert shouting about "saving America." Save your marriage instead. The world doesn't need more angry voters—it needs more satisfied lovers. Politics divides: passion unites.

Forget the polls. Forget the pundits. The only campaign worth fighting for is the one that begins in your bedroom.

Make peace. Make love. Make America Mate Again.

Comme on dit en France:
L'amour est la seule politique qui mérite votre vote.

As we say in France:
Love is the only politics worth voting for.

About the Author

Guy Blaise is a French author whose work bridges the cultural gap between passion and reason, intimacy and independence. After living in both France and the United States, he began observing the emotional and romantic disconnect that too often defines modern relationships. His mission became clear: to reintroduce the art of love- the French way-into American bedrooms.

Blending empathy, humor and candor, Blaise writes about unspoken struggle couples face and how to rekindle desire without losing dignity. His bold, poetic reflections have resonated with readers seeking truth over trends and depth over performance. He is also the author of Love Like the French, and when he is not writing, he divides his time between cafes, long runs and conversations that still believe in love and precious moments with his daughters who remind him why love-in all its forms- is worth fighting for.

www.ingramcontent.com/pod-product-compliance
Lightning Source LLC
LaVergne TN
LVHW021740050126
829120LV00017B/1525